THE ESSENTIAL BOY'S GUIDE TO PUBERTY & BODY CHANGES, AGES 8-14

UNDERSTAND YOUR BODY, EMBRACE THE CHANGES
& GROW-UP WITH CONFIDENCE

DEBBIEANN LEWIS

CONTENTS

Introduction   5

1. Welcome to the Adventure—Understanding Puberty Your Way   9
2. Body Glow-Up—What Changes and Why   27
3. Hygiene Heroes—Mastering the Basics Without the Lecture   43
4. Brainwaves & Mood Swings—Your Changing Mind and Emotions   59
5. Squad Goals—Friendships, Teasing, and Social Superpowers   77
6. Fuel, Rest, and Strength—Taking Care of Your Changing Body   95
7. Real Talk Q&A—Honest Answers to Your Toughest Questions   113
8. Confidence, Consent & Kindness—Growing Into the Best Version of You   133

Conclusion   151
Glossary of Terms   157
References   161

INTRODUCTION

Let's be honest: nothing prepares you for the day your voice squeaks in the middle of class. Or the moment you realize your favorite T-shirt smells like a locker room, even though you "totally" remembered deodorant (or did you?). Puberty can show up out of nowhere and make things awkward, confusing, and sometimes a little embarrassing. Whether it's worrying about growing taller, hair popping up in new places, or just feeling like your body is suddenly running its own secret program, it can all feel pretty weird.

I know this because I've seen it up close. I'm DebbieAnn—a mom of four, a grandmother of five, and someone who has spent years talking with kids and parents about bodies, growing up, and all the stuff nobody wants to ask out loud. I have heard the questions, the worries, and the funny stories. I've watched boys try to act cool when they're secretly wondering if everyone else is feeling just as weird as they are (spoiler: yes, they are).

I wrote this book because, honestly, there are not enough books that talk to you—really talk to you—about what's going on. The books at school? Usually too scientific, too boring, or all about girls. The stuff you find online? Sometimes helpful, sometimes confusing, and sometimes just plain wrong. Most resources leave boys' worries hanging in the air. Questions like: "Is this normal?" "Will anyone notice?" or "Am I the only one?" don't always get answered.

That's not okay with me. You deserve straight answers, real talk, and some actual help. My vision for this book is simple. I want it to be the kind of guide I wish every boy could have. One that makes you feel less alone. One that helps you laugh at the weird stuff, find answers to the awkward stuff, and know you're not the only one going through it.

Think of this book as a big brother, a coach, or a really honest friend who's been down this road before. I promise not to lecture. No one needs another boring class or a list of rules. Instead, I'll give you real advice, stories from other boys, and tips that actually make sense. I want you to feel comfortable flipping through these pages, whether you're reading by yourself or with someone you trust.

You matter, exactly as you are. Boys come in all shapes, sizes, backgrounds, and families. This book is for all of you. It doesn't matter if you're the tallest in class or still waiting to grow, if you live with one parent, two grandparents, or a whole crew. Every boy should see himself in these pages and know he belongs.

So, what are we going to talk about? Everything you need to know to get through puberty, like feeling strong, confident, and yes—even a little more chill about the whole thing. We'll cover what happens to your body (and why it's not as scary as you think). We'll talk about hygiene (because smelling good is always a win). We'll look at emotions (yes, even the ones that sneak up on you). We'll talk about friendships, school, digital life, and how to handle the stuff that makes you want to scream into a pillow. Most of all, we'll talk about growing into a kind, respectful, and confident guy.

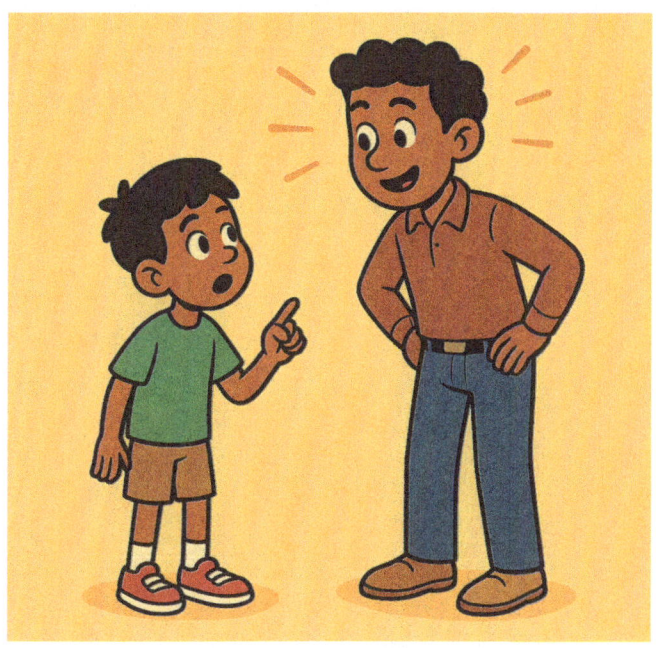

And here's a secret: this book isn't just for you. It's also for the people who care about you—parents, grandparents, teachers, coaches, and anyone else who wants to help you along the way. You can hand them this book if you're not sure how to start a conversation. Or you can read it on your own and surprise them with all the stuff you've learned. Either way, it's a tool for everyone.

I know you might have questions you're too embarrassed to ask out loud. Things about body changes, hair, sweat, crushes, or feeling different. Maybe you're worried you're behind or ahead of your friends. Maybe you wonder if something weird is happening only to you. No question is too strange, too silly, or too private.

I've heard them all, and I promise to answer them as honestly as I can. You don't have to figure this stuff out alone.

So here's my invitation to you: let's go through this together. Puberty doesn't have to be something you dread. It can be a journey—a little weird, a little wild, but also full of growth and discovery. You might even surprise yourself with how strong, kind, and confident you become.

Ready? Let's get started. You've got this.

1

WELCOME TO THE ADVENTURE— UNDERSTANDING PUBERTY YOUR WAY

Ever been sitting in class, minding your own business, and suddenly, your voice decides to squeak like a rusty door hinge? Or maybe you're running around at recess, and you notice your shirt is a little damp under your arms—even though you barely broke a sweat last year. If you've had one of these moments, you're not alone. I remember watching one of my sons try to call for the family dog, only to hear his voice crack so loudly the dog actually stopped in his tracks. He went red as a tomato, but here's the thing: after laughing it off, he realized even his friends had their own "squeaky" stories.

This chapter is all about figuring out what's really happening. Puberty feels like a secret level in a video game that you didn't even know existed. Suddenly, new powers and surprises keep popping up, and there's no guidebook that makes sense until now. My goal is to make this feel less like a pop quiz and more like having a backstage pass where you get the inside scoop—no fluff, no boring lectures.

REAL TALK—WHAT PUBERTY ACTUALLY MEANS (NO CAP!)

Let's start with the basics. Puberty is just a fancy word for when your body decides it's time to grow up. Think of it as leveling up in real life. All these changes might seem random at first, but they actually mean your body is getting stronger, taller, and more grown-up. It's like unlocking new skills in a game—one day, you're just you, and the next day, you might have new hair on your legs or feel hungry all the time. You might even notice you suddenly care about things like how your breath smells or if your skin is clear.

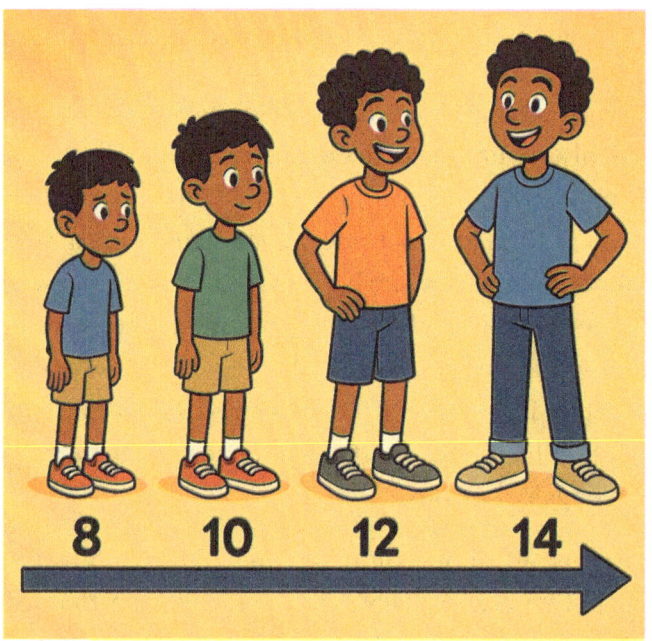

As this "level up" begins, you'll spot a bunch of changes—some big, some small, and some just plain weird. Growth spurts can hit fast; you might wake up one day and realize your pants seem way shorter than yesterday. You might get hair in places where there wasn't hair before—like under your arms, above your lip, or even on your legs. This can feel shocking at first, but everyone goes through it. Your skin might get oily or break out with pimples. Sometimes, you'll sweat more than before, even if you're not running around outside. Your voice might bounce from high to low like it's trying out for a singing contest. There are days when emotions feel bigger, too—you could be happy one moment and then annoyed or sad for no reason.

Every boy, everywhere, goes through this, no matter where they live or what they look like. You might think, "Nobody else is dealing with this," but trust me, they are. Jalen in Florida wonders why his feet grew two sizes in one summer. Ethan in Oregon is the first in his squad to need deodorant and feels weird about it. Mateo in Texas started getting a mustache before any of his friends did. Samir in New York sometimes feels embarrassed because he cries at sad movies now when before he never did. These stories are normal and happen to everyone, even if they don't talk about them. Puberty isn't just for one type of boy—it happens to all boys everywhere.

This book is your safe zone. Nothing is too strange or off-limits here. You can treat these pages like having a private coach who always tells the truth—or maybe like having a super chill older brother who has already survived this stage and wants to help you out. You'll find answers to the awkward stuff your friends whisper about but never ask out loud. You'll get real advice that actually works in real life—not just in a science class or from some boring slideshow at school.

No question is a dumb question here. If you wonder about something—like why your armpits suddenly smell different, like raw onions, or why you feel angry for no reason—it's fair game. If you want to know how to handle teasing or what to say to parents when things get weird, you'll find those tips, too. I promise I'll answer as honestly as possible because everybody deserves answers that make sense—not answers that make you feel more confused.

Try This: Your Own "Level Up" Checklist

Let's make this fun. Grab a notebook or use the space below to write down any new things you notice about yourself this year—maybe you started using deodorant, noticed your voice dropped a little, or had your first growth spurt. Every time something new pops up, add it to your list and give yourself a high-five for unlocking another skill. It's not about keeping score with anyone else; it's just about tracking how far you've come.

Puberty brings changes all over—body, mind, and emotions—but you're not alone or weird for feeling unsure about it all. Treat this book as your go-to playbook where nothing is too awkward or embarrassing to ask.

WHY EVERYONE'S TIMELINE IS DIFFERENT (AND THAT'S NORMAL)

Ever wondered why some boys need to shave early while others still look like their third-grade photos? Or how you might shoot up a few inches in a summer while your friends barely grow? Puberty isn't a synchronized event—it's more like a bus that picks people up at different stops, with everyone boarding at their own pace. There's no way to control when your "ticket" is punched, and nothing's wrong if you're early or late.

Science backs this up: puberty can start anywhere from age nine to fourteen. Genes play a big part—if your family members developed late or early, you might too. But it's not just genetics; your

WELCOME TO THE ADVENTURE—UNDERSTANDING PUBERT... | 13

diet, activity, stress, sleep, and general health all help decide your body's schedule.

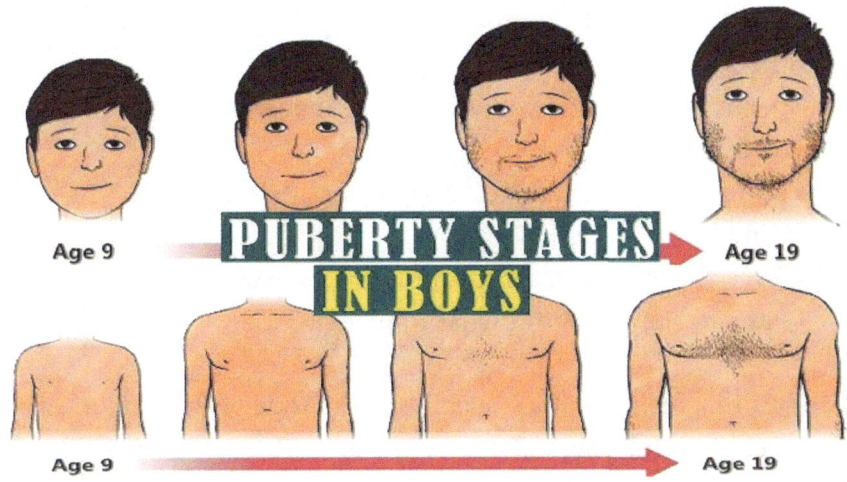

Picture Marcus and Leo, best friends who eat the same food and play the same games. After winter break, Marcus is suddenly taller, speaks deeper, and is into hair gel. Leo still looks and feels the same and wonders if he's behind. Actually, Marcus's body just hit the "grow" button sooner. Leo's changes will come in time—both are right on track.

It's perfectly normal to feel out of place if your body seems "off schedule." Maybe you're anxious about being the last to change, or you wish changes weren't happening so soon. Comparing yourself to classmates is common, but it only makes you feel worse. Puberty isn't a contest; there's no prize for finishing first or last.

If you find yourself worrying or comparing, remember that every timeline is normal. Most boys begin puberty between ages nine and fourteen, and there's no "correct" order for changes. You can't lose points for being early or late.

Here's a quick checklist—are you caught in the "comparison trap"?

- Do you constantly compare your height or body to others?
- Spend more energy worrying about appearances than how you feel?
- Feel upset if your changes are quicker or slower than friends?
- Check the mirror every morning for signs of change?
- Listen to rumors about what's "normal"?

If any of this feels familiar, take a breath. Your body is on a timeline that's right for you.

Let's Try: The Comparison Buster

The next time you notice you're comparing yourself:

1. Think of one thing you like about yourself right now—even if it has nothing to do with your body.
2. Remember, everyone wants something about themselves to change—faster or slower.
3. Remind yourself that nobody— not even twins—grows at exactly the same rate.
4. Celebrate a small achievement, like scoring in a game or making someone laugh.

Remember: bodies come in all shapes, sizes, and shades. Some boys get broad shoulders early, others later; some grow tall fast and then fill out, and others do both at once. Traits such as skin color, hair texture, height, and build are inherited from your family and your unique combination of traits. You might be tall

WELCOME TO THE ADVENTURE—UNDERSTANDING PUBERT... | 15

and thin, short and strong, or anywhere in between—all perfectly normal.

Look around your school, and you'll see this in action: Malik grows taller than everyone later on, Diego is short, but the fastest runner, Aiden's mustache shows up before anyone else's, and Kai adds muscle before needing to shave. Everyone's story is different—and that's how it should be.

Instead of keeping score, try tracking your own milestones. Maybe your voice stays low for a whole sentence, or someone notices your strength (even if it's just carrying groceries). Give yourself credit for your unique steps forward whenever they happen.

If you're worried about your timing or can't shake the feeling that something's wrong, talk to a parent or another adult you trust. Most things you feel awkward admitting are completely normal. Everyone's pace is unique—and that's what makes growing up interesting, not scary.

BUSTING MYTH #1: THERE'S NO "PERFECT" AGE FOR PUBERTY

Think about the rumors you hear at school. Maybe someone said, "If you don't have armpit hair by sixth grade, something's wrong." Or perhaps a friend told you that everyone should start puberty at the same age, or you're behind if your voice still sounds the same as it did in third grade. Here's the truth: there is no magic age where everyone's body flips the switch. That idea? Total myth. Puberty does not show up with a schedule that fits all boys. If you ask ten guys when their changes started, you'll get ten different answers—and all of them are normal.

Some boys might notice their bodies changing at eight or nine. Others might not see much happening until twelve, thirteen, or even fourteen. Doctors examine a vast age range and consider it all normal. You could be the first in your class to shoot up a few inches, or you could still look like your old school photo while your friends are suddenly taller. Neither is better or worse. It's just your personal timing. In fact, most kids start somewhere between nine and fourteen years old, but there are plenty of outliers.

Imagine a comic strip panel:

Kid A has a mustache shadow at eleven,
Kid B is still wearing the same shoe size at thirteen,
Kid C gets taller at ten,
Kid D's voice doesn't crack until almost high school.

Every path works.

Let's highlight some stats and fun facts to make it real. Starting puberty at eight is rare, but it is possible. Ten is common—lots of boys notice things changing around this time. Twelve is also pretty average. For some, thirteen is when things begin. All of these fit within what doctors expect for healthy growth. There is no "winner" or "loser" here. No one gets a trophy for being first.

Let's do a quick Q&A to clear up more of those silent worries:

- **Q: Is something wrong with me if nothing has changed yet?**
    - **A**: *Not at all. Doctors see a wide range of ages and call them all healthy. You're not left behind—you're just waiting for your turn.*
- **Q: My friend already has a deep voice, and I don't. Is that bad?**
    - **A**: *Totally fine. Voices drop at different times for everyone.*

- **Q: What if I'm first?**
  - A: *That's normal too! Some boys lead the pack, and some follow later.*
- **Q: Can I speed things up or slow them down?**
  - A: *Not really—your body sets its own plan, and that's best for you.*

Rumors will always buzz around school, but remember they're just that—rumors. You can't "miss" puberty, and you can't do it wrong.

Instead of looking at other people and checking off who's ahead or behind, try focusing on your own progress. This isn't a race, and there are no gold medals for crossing some imaginary finish line first. Remember, even best friends won't hit every change at the same time.

It's easy to feel pressure from what you see in the locker room or hear online, especially when people act like there's some perfect checklist for growing up. Don't let that stress creep in. Every boy's path looks different. Some bodies change early, some wait longer—and that's how it should be. You can trust your body to do its thing when it's ready.

CHOOSE-YOUR-PATH: YOU VS. THE AWKWARD STAGE

Ever felt like your body was playing tricks on you just for laughs? It's like your body's sense of humor makes you the punchline. Welcome to the "awkward stage." But it's not a curse—it's a common experience, something everyone, even the "cool" kids, parents, and teachers, go through. Ask anyone, and they'll have their own cringe story from when they wanted to melt into their hoodie.

Take my son, for instance: he once came down for breakfast with his hair sticking up like a rooster. He wandered around for an hour that way, then laughed and slapped some water on his head when he finally saw himself in a mirror. That's a perfect example—surviving the awkward stage means laughing it off and realizing it's hardly the end of the world.

Choose-Your-Path Game

Let's put you in the spotlight with a "choose-your-path" game.

You're in science class, a quiz is coming, and your teacher calls your name. You start to answer, but your voice cracks loudly.

What do you do?

- A. Freeze and wish for invisibility.
- B. Joke about turning into a robot.
- C. Finish your answer and pretend nothing happened.

If you **pick A?**, you're normal—everyone freezes sometimes, but it passes quickly. **B?** Great—using humor relaxes the room, and **C?** works too—just pushing forward lets the moment pass. Whichever you pick, the moment barely lasts, and by lunchtime, nobody remembers.

Here's another scenario: Playing basketball after school, you spot big sweat stains under your arms.

- A. Try to hide them by crossing your arms the rest of the game.
- B. Point them out and say, "Guess I'm working hard out here!"
- C. Ask a friend for a spare shirt.

Each choice is valid. Hiding only works for so long, humor shows confidence, and asking for help shows you trust your friends—rarely do people want to tease you for it.

Embarrassing moments feel huge in the moment but shrink quickly, and those self-conscious feelings are temporary. If you could hear everyone's thoughts, you'd realize how many people worry about their own "**weird**" moments.

Here are a couple of *"Awkward Wins"* from real boys who survived their most cringe-worthy moments. One boy's stomach growled so loudly in math that everyone looked over—he shrugged and said, "Yikes, I skipped breakfast." Everyone laughed, and several others admitted they were hungry too. Another boy tripped while getting an award at assembly, bowed, and got extra applause.

When awkward things happen—like a joke about your body odor or a comment about a zit—you can bounce back faster than you think. Try these tips:

- **Laugh it off:** "Guess my superpower is clearing rooms!" or "Good thing showers exist, right?" Humor removes the sting.
- **Self-talk**: Remind yourself that awkward moments happen to everyone.
- **Practice what to say**:
    - "Yeah, puberty is wild."
    - "Happens to everyone."
    - "It's just a phase—I'll survive."
    - "Aren't you glad that happened to me, not you?"

Feeling like everyone's staring can be tough, but it rarely lasts. Here's a quick checklist for those moments:

What To Do When You Feel Like Everyone's Staring

- Take a deep breath.
- Remind yourself: "This will pass."
- Find a friendly face, or focus on someone who isn't paying attention.
- Concentrate on your next step, not what just happened.
- Give yourself credit for handling it.

The awkward stage is just part of growing up, not a reason to shy away or feel bad about yourself. One day, these moments will become funny stories and reminders that you can handle whatever life throws at you—even when things get weird.

GROWTH TRACKERS & FIRSTS—CELEBRATING YOUR UNIQUE MILESTONES

Puberty can feel random, but it's actually full of "firsts" that are worth remembering. Instead of thinking of each new thing as a problem, what if you flipped it? Imagine you're collecting achievements, like in a video game or on a sports team. The first time you use deodorant—achievement is unlocked! The first time you spot a tiny shadow above your lip—a new badge has been earned! These moments are like hidden trophies, and you're the only one who gets to decide how cool they are. Some boys might keep score in their heads, and others might just smile at themselves. No matter how you do it, your milestones matter.

You don't need a big crowd to celebrate. Sometimes, the best celebrations are those that are quiet. You can slip yourself a high-five behind closed doors or scribble a note in your notebook: "Today, my voice sounded deeper on the phone." Some guys like to draw a funny cartoon or sketch a quick doodle to mark the moment.

WELCOME TO THE ADVENTURE—UNDERSTANDING PUBERT... | 21

Maybe you even want to write a secret code in your calendar for the day you tried cologne for the first time. It's your adventure, your way.

Physical changes receive a lot of attention, but that's not the whole story. Sure, you'll notice things like taller legs or new hair, but think about other "firsts" too. The first time you stand up for a friend who's getting teased is huge. Telling an adult how you really feel is a new skill, like learning how to ride a bike without hands. Even deciding to take care of your skin or making your own breakfast are milestones. These count just as much as the body stuff.

Nobody else's timeline matters here; it's all about what feels important to you. If you want, try making your own "Growth Tracker" right in this book or ask someone for a printable page. Here's an idea for your tracker: draw boxes next to each "first," then fill them in as they happen.

Examples:

Growth Tracker

- ☐ First deodorant
- ☐ First growth spurt
- ☐ First pimple
- ☐ First deeper voice day
- ☐ First time talking about feelings
- ☐ First time helping someone else
- ☐ First time admitting you were wrong
- ☐ First time handling your own laundry
- ☐
- ☐
- ☐

Every box you check is a win. You can create and add your own badges or stickers for these moments, too. Give yourself permission to add anything that matters—even if it seems small to someone else. Every checked box is proof that you are leveling up in your own way, at your own speed.

If you want to keep it private, write down only what matters most to you. Some boys never show anyone their tracker; others might share it with a parent, grandparent, or even a friend who gets it.

If you're into journaling, try this: after something new happens—big or small—take five minutes to jot down what happened and how it made you feel. Maybe you felt proud or embarrassed or just plain surprised. There's no right answer. You can even sketch what happened if drawing feels easier than writing.

Think about the first time you decided not to laugh at someone else's awkward moment and instead checked if they were okay. That's a milestone, too, and it says a lot about the kind of person you're growing into. Or maybe you said "no" when someone pressured you to do something that felt wrong. These emotional and social wins deserve badges right beside your physical changes.

You might not realize it yet, but tracking these moments helps you see how much you've grown—not just on the outside but inside, too. Years from now, you'll look back at your lists or notes and remember when everything felt new and weird. You'll see how each first shaped who you are becoming. Some days will feel slow, with nothing changing at all, while others will surprise you with two achievements in one afternoon.

If you want some ideas for celebrating these wins, here are a few: treat yourself to your favorite snack, play your favorite song extra loud in your room, or just pause and think, "Nice job." Some boys like to give themselves a silly nickname for the day, like "Captain

Fresh Breath," after trying mouthwash for the first time. Others might invent their own handshake and do it solo—who cares if it looks goofy? It's your badge.

Remember, this is not about showing off or making anyone else feel bad. It's about noticing what makes your story special. Your body and mind will both hit new levels over time, and each milestone deserves its own little moment of celebration.

GOT ANXIETY? WHY FEELING WEIRD IS TOTALLY COMMON

Waking up and feeling like a stranger in your own skin, catching your reflection and wondering what's changed, or worrying about things that didn't used to bother you—like your height, asking questions in class, or whether others are handling life better—are all super normal when your body and brain are changing. Feeling weird, worried, or a bit lost is just part of growing up.

Puberty often magnifies every emotion. One minute, you're laughing; the next, you're suddenly quiet or uneasy, without knowing why. It can be confusing, even scary, but it's simply your brain running a major "software update." Like a phone acting up after a big update, your brain is rewiring, making new connections, and handling a surge of hormones. That's why your emotions can swing wildly—you might feel awesome, then awkward, then anxious, all before lunch.

These feelings don't mean anything is wrong; they're just signs your brain and body are working hard to grow up. Hormones like testosterone send mixed signals, making you feel jumpy, hungry, emotional, or wanting to be alone. Worrying about being "normal" is a fairly typical part of this stage.

New worries might start to show up—"What if I never catch up?" "Why do I feel different every day?" Or you might begin stressing about things you never thought of before: how you smell after gym, your voice, or if your friends notice you acting differently. These thoughts can pile up, making you tense or nervous.

The good news is that there are ways to handle anxious and weird feelings so they don't take over your day. Sometimes, simple tricks can make a big difference. When worries get overwhelming, slow things down by taking deep breaths—in through your nose, out through your mouth. Try counting to five as you breathe in and five as you breathe out. This calms your body and reassures your brain.

Keeping your worries in check can help. When anxious thoughts pop up (like, "Everyone is staring at me!"), answer back with something positive, even if it feels weird: "This will pass," or "Everyone feels weird sometimes." You can also jot thoughts down or draw what your anxiety looks like—a tangle, a storm cloud, whatever comes to mind. Seeing it on paper can make the feeling seem smaller.

Sometimes, drawing helps more than talking. Grab a pencil and sketch what anxiety feels like—a scribble, a circle, anything. The point is just to get the feelings out of your head for a bit.

Chill-Out Checklist

- Take five deep breaths.
- Move to a quiet place if things feel overwhelming.
- Squeeze a stress ball or stretch your hands.
- Have a drink of water.
- Remind yourself: "This won't last forever."

- Think of one thing you did well today, even if it's something small.

Almost everyone feels anxious or awkward sometimes, even if they never mention it. Some are afraid they'll never fit in, others just want a break from their busy thoughts. You're not alone. If the feelings stick around or feel too big, talk to someone who can help—don't keep it to yourself. You don't have to handle this alone. Trusted adults—parents, grandparents, siblings, teachers, counselors, or coaches—are there to listen, even if it feels hard to start the conversation. If talking is tough, try writing your feelings down first.

Everyone has weird days—including adults who seem cool on the outside. Puberty shakes things up for everyone. What's most important is realizing these feelings are normal and learning to handle them.

If you want, use journal prompts to jot down what's bothering you or what helps you on tough days. Sometimes, seeing your thoughts in writing makes them less overwhelming.

No matter how strange or unpredictable things feel now, you're not the only one feeling this way. Every day is a step forward, and there are always people ready to help if you need them.

2

BODY GLOW-UP—WHAT CHANGES AND WHY

WHY YOUR BODY'S GROWING IN FUNNY WAYS (HELLO, GROWTH SPURTS!)

Sometimes, you wake up, and your bed feels smaller. Your toes push against the end of the footboard or hang off the end of the mattress, and you wonder if your bed shrank overnight. But nope—it's just you. Growth spurts do not play around. One week, your pants fit fine; the next, you have "high-waters" that show off your socks. It can be a shock when your favorite hoodie feels tight around the arms or you suddenly need new shoes because your big toe is poking out. Growth spurts are one of the most classic signs puberty has hit, and they never seem to arrive quietly.

A growth spurt is a period when your body grows much faster than usual. For boys, this usually starts somewhere between ages nine and fourteen, but everyone's clock is different. Some guys shoot up early and seem like giants in middle school. Others grow later and catch up in high school. Take Jayden, who hit his growth spurt in fourth grade. He went from being the shortest kid in class to looking over everyone's heads by the end of fifth grade. His mom bought new jeans every three months, and he kept bumping his knee on his desk because he was not used to his longer legs. Then there's Eli, who waited and waited while his friends grew taller. He wondered if he'd ever stretch out. Finally, in eighth grade, Eli shot up almost six inches in one summer. He remembers lying on the couch with sore knees and eating cereal from the giant bowl. Both boys felt awkward at first, but both ended up right where they needed to be.

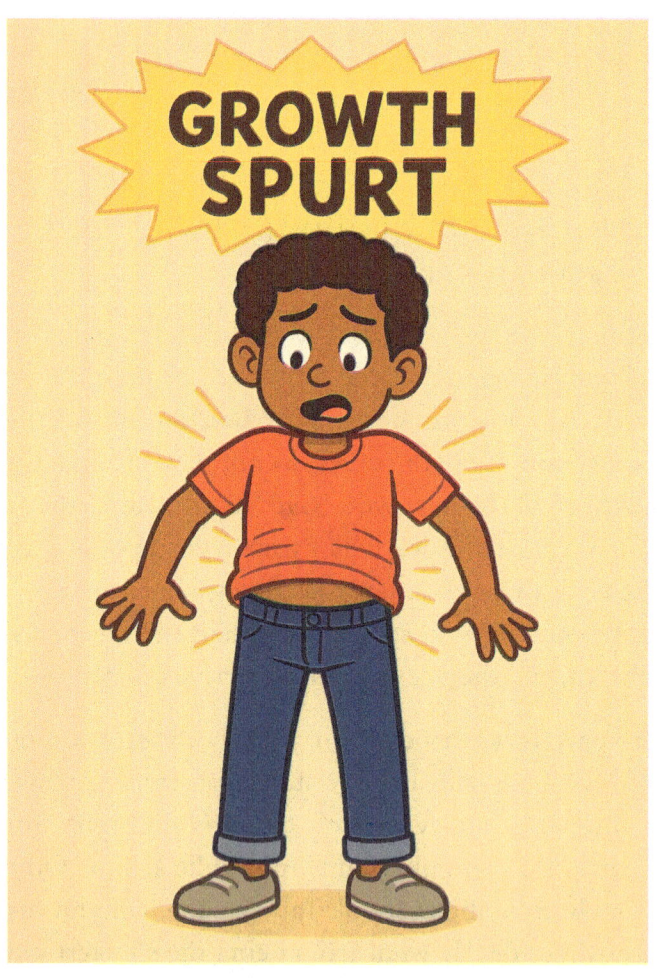

Growth spurts can feel sudden and strange. You might notice your wrists and ankles get bigger before anything else does. Your shirts feel tight in the shoulders, or you keep tripping over things you used to step over easily. Some boys grow so quickly that their shoes wear out at the toes before the rest even looks old. You might even need a new bed if your feet start hanging off the end every night! These changes are normal—even if they make you feel like a clumsy baby giraffe learning how to walk for the first time.

The body works hard during a growth spurt. You might feel tired more often or get really hungry out of nowhere. Some days, you want to eat everything in the fridge, then go back for seconds. This is because your body needs extra fuel to handle all that building and stretching. Your bones are growing longer, your muscles are getting stronger, and everything is working extra hard to catch up. You might also feel aches in your knees, shins, or back. These "growing pains" can make it tough to fall asleep or get comfy on the couch.

Feeling clumsy is part of the deal. Your arms and legs grow so fast that sometimes your brain needs time to catch up. It's totally normal to knock over a glass of milk or misjudge a doorway and bump your shoulder. I once watched my own grandson try to sit at his regular spot at the dinner table, but his legs were suddenly taller than last week as he was knocking his knees. He looked surprised, then laughed it off as his "giraffe move." It happens to everyone at least once.

When you're growing quick, it helps to take care of yourself in small ways. Gentle stretching can ease some of those aches. Try reaching up high with both hands or doing slow toe-touches before bed or after you wake up. Drinking enough water can help, too—your body needs it for building muscle and bone. Make sure you eat foods with protein, calcium, and vitamins. That means things like eggs, chicken, beans, cheese, milk, yogurt, or even a handful of almonds if you like nuts. And while it sounds simple, sleeping enough is huge for growth. Your body does most of its building at night while you sleep.

If you notice increased tiredness after a week of rapid growth, listen to your body and rest when you can. Don't be surprised if you need an afternoon nap or feel sleepy earlier than usual some days.

Quick Checklist: Handling Your Growth Spurt Like a Pro

- Stretch before bed and after waking up.
- Eat snacks with protein and calcium.
- Drink water during the day.
- Rest when you feel tired.
- Laugh off clumsy moments (bonus points for style).

It's easy to feel off-balance during a growth spurt, but remember: every boy goes through this in his own way and at his own speed. One day, you're bumping into tables or tripping over your feet; soon enough, your brain catches up, and you'll feel more coordinated again. Each step (even the clumsy ones) means your body is getting stronger and ready for whatever comes next.

HAIR HERE, THERE, EVERYWHERE—WHAT'S UP WITH NEW HAIR?

During puberty, one of the most noticeable changes is the sudden appearance of new body hair. It can seem like your body is starting a secret garden, as soft hair appears under your arms, on your legs, face, or around your groin. Some boys notice thicker or darker hair in certain areas first, while others see just a few curly hairs at first. Timing and appearance are different for everyone—your body hair might be fine, dark, light, curly, straight, or any combination, and how it grows is affected by your genes. There's no "normal" look or schedule; body hair can show up early for some boys and later for others, even within the same family.

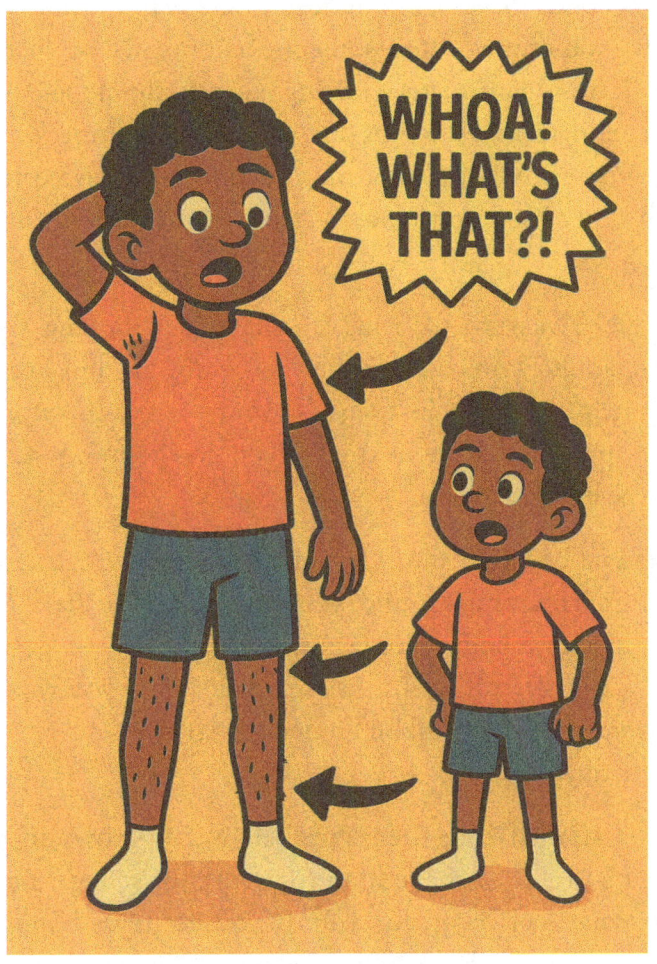

Questions like, "Why is my armpit hair darker than my arm hair?" or "How come my friend has a mustache but I don't?" are common. The answer is simple: everyone follows their own pattern. Some guys see leg hair first, others notice a shadow on their lip; someone might be shaving at fifteen while another still has barely-there fuzz at the same age. The hair on your face or underarms can grow in a different color or texture than your head hair—even siblings often have totally different body hair.

When new hair appears, you might wonder what to do. There aren't rules about shaving or trimming—many boys wait until they feel ready, sometimes after someone comments or just out of curiosity. If you want to try shaving, keep it simple and safe: use shaving cream (not just soap) and choose a beginner's razor or electric trimmer. Ask a parent or someone experienced for guidance, and don't hesitate to watch instructional videos together if you need help.

It might feel awkward to bring up shaving or buying your first razor, but adults know it's part of growing up and are usually happy to help. You can just say, "I want to try shaving," or ask about picking out a razor next time you go shopping—there's no reason to be embarrassed.

Good hygiene becomes more important with new hair, especially under your arms and around your groin, where hair can trap sweat and increase body odor. Shower regularly, wash gently with soap and water, dry off well, and use deodorant if you want. If you shave, always rinse the razor after each stroke, and never share razors with anyone else.

Some boys start styling their facial hair if it grows in enough, while others prefer to shave it all for sports or school. There's no rush—do what feels right for you. If you get teased about being "hairy" or not having much hair, remember that everyone's body is different, and hair will show up in its own time.

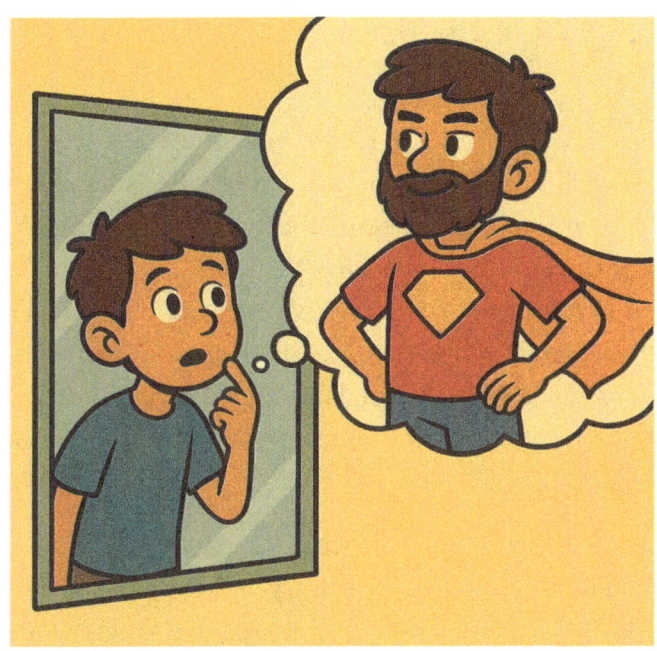

Some friends might be excited to grow a mustache, while others wish their leg hair would stay away longer. Either way, body hair simply means you're growing up—at your own pace. Don't let others pressure you to shave before you want to-or make you feel weird if you don't want to shave yet.

THE GREAT VOICE CRACK & WHY IT HAPPENS

You open your mouth to answer a question in class, and your voice suddenly jumps from deep to high like a cartoon character. Maybe you're telling a joke, and in the middle of your best line, your voice cracks so hard that you have to laugh. This is the classic voice change, and it happens to every boy during puberty. There is nothing quite like it. Sometimes, your voice sounds low and grown-up, then, out of nowhere, it squeaks or wobbles like a sound effect. You might worry everyone will stare, but the truth is, most people have been through it themselves. Even adult men remember their own "voice crack" days.

What's really going on here? Inside your neck is a part called the larynx, or voice box. Before puberty, this spot is small and keeps your voice light and high. When puberty kicks in, your body sends out new hormones, and the larynx grows bigger and stronger. Your vocal cords inside the larynx stretch out and thicken. Think of this as a voice upgrade—like getting a new speaker that suddenly has more bass. As the larynx gets bigger, you can sometimes see a bump form at the front of your throat. That's called an Adam's apple, and it's a sign your voice is changing for good.

While the larynx grows, your vocal cords need time to adjust. They don't always move smoothly yet. This is why your voice might squeak, crack, or shift without warning. One day, you might sound deep and smooth. The next day, you sound like you swallowed a kazoo. That's normal! Some boys get voice cracks once in a while, and others get them every day for months. Sometimes, it happens during a big school presentation or when you yell at recess. The sound can be funny—a mix between a whistle and a hiccup—and yes, it's easy to feel embarrassed when it happens in public.

There was a time when my own son was reading aloud in class, and halfway through his sentence, his voice cracked so loud his teacher stopped to check if he was okay. He turned red, but the teacher just smiled and said, "Puberty's here!" Another boy I know was singing at his cousin's birthday party when his voice squeaked mid-song. Everyone giggled, but he just grinned and kept on singing. These moments feel huge when they happen, but they're actually quick and forgettable for everyone else.

If your voice cracks in front of others, try to keep it light and relaxed. You can shrug it off with a joke like, "Oops, puberty in progress!" or "My voice didn't get the memo today." Most people will laugh with you because they get it—or they remember their own voice-crack horror stories. Don't panic or feel like you need to hide. It helps to talk about it with friends or older siblings who have been through it already. They'll probably have stories that are even funnier than yours.

Remember that all this weirdness is temporary. Your body is just sorting out how to use its new "voice gear." Over time, things settle down. Your voice gets lower and steadier. The cracks typically fade away, usually after about six months to a year, although this can sometimes take longer for some boys. Every person's timeline is different, but everyone makes it through.

If you ever feel nervous about an upcoming speech or presentation, practice reading out loud at home first. If your voice cracks while practicing, just keep going. The more you talk with your new, deeper voice, the faster your vocal cords settle into their new job. Drink water to keep your throat comfortable—sometimes a dry mouth makes cracks worse.

Here are a few more tips for owning your voice cracks:

- Don't try to force your voice lower on purpose. Let it find its own level.
- Laugh off the awkward moments; humor always wins.
- If someone teases you, remember they'll probably be cracking soon, too (or already have).

Most important of all, don't let a silly crack hold you back from speaking up or sharing your ideas. Your real friends will remember what you said—not how it sounded for two seconds.

Voice changes are one of those classic markers of puberty that everyone experiences in their own way. It's kind of like a badge that proves you're growing up—even if it makes you sound like a broken robot now and then. So when your voice does its glitchy dance at the worst possible moment, just roll with it. You're not alone in this; you're just getting upgraded, one squeak at a time.

BREAKOUTS, ZITS, AND SKIN SURPRISES—DEALING WITH ACNE

One day, you look in the mirror, and, bam, there's a red bump on your forehead. Or maybe you wake up with little dots on your nose or a sore chin. You're not turning into an alien—this is acne. It shows up for almost everyone during puberty because changing hormones rev up your oil glands. Oil keeps skin healthy, but too much mixes with dead skin and blocks pores. When that happens, you get pimples or blackheads. Blame hormones and genes, not being dirty, or that one slice of pizza.

There are different types of bumps. Blackheads are small dark dots —that open at the top, turning dark when the air hits the oil inside. Whiteheads are closed bumps with a white tip. Regular pimples get red, swollen, and sometimes sore. Deeper, painful bumps are called cysts. You might get one big pimple, or a bunch together. Most boys get some acne, especially if it runs in the family.

Many myths about acne only make things worse. You might hear that only people who don't wash get pimples or that chocolate or potato chips cause zits. Actually, over-washing can dry out the skin and trigger more oil. For most people, acne is about hormones, not what they eat. Popping a zit won't help either—squeezing pushes bacteria deeper and can cause scars that last longer than the spot.

Myth-Buster Callout: True or False—Does Pizza Cause Pimples?

False! Eating pizza or chocolate occasionally won't cause a breakout. For most people, pimples come from changes inside, not a single snack.

Taking care of your skin doesn't need to be complicated.

Keep your routine simple:

- Wash gently twice a day (morning and night) using warm water and a mild cleanser. Avoid gritty or harsh products.
- Rinse well and pat dry—don't rub or scrub at pimples.
- After sweating, wash your face to keep pores clear.
- Never share towels or facecloths; bacteria can spread that way.

Try not to pop or pick at pimples. Picking spreads germs and can scar. Use hair products carefully, keeping them away from your forehead, and wash your hair regularly since some products can clog pores.

Sometimes, breakouts persist no matter what you do. If gentle washing isn't enough and you get lots of red bumps or painful cysts, ask for help. Talk to an adult about using special creams or visiting a doctor. Sometimes stronger creams or medicines help when regular routines don't. There's no shame in needing a little extra help—skin can be stubborn during puberty.

If you ever feel upset about your skin or get teased, remember: everyone gets acne at some point, even celebrities and "cool" kids. You're not alone, and it will get better as you grow up. A little patience helps. Some days will be bumpier than others, but stick with what works and ignore wild skincare fads online. Your skin's doing its job while you grow up—no filter required.

"IS THIS NORMAL?"—WHEN ONE PART GROWS FASTER THAN THE REST

It's wild how your body seems to be working off its own secret blueprint during puberty. You might wake up and notice your feet look way too long for your legs or that your hands seem to belong to somebody bigger. Maybe you look in the mirror and realize your nose looks a bit different, or your arms seem out of place on your body. It's easy to wonder if something is off.

You might even ask, "Why do I have feet the size of flippers but still a small frame?" This feeling is so common, even though nobody really talks about it. I remember watching my son, who suddenly had "baseball mitt" hands but was still a skinny kid. He would try to grip a basketball, and it looked like he was wearing clown gloves compared to the year before. He was embarrassed for a while, worried that everyone would notice, but in a year, his arms and shoulders had caught up, and he was back to feeling balanced.

Science indicates that this uneven growth is entirely normal. Your body doesn't grow all at once; it builds in stages, much like upgrading a character in a video game. First, one part levels up, then another. Your feet and hands usually grow first, then your arms and legs. The rest of your body catches up later. This process can leave you feeling mismatched for a bit—like you're wearing shoes too big for your body or like your sleeves are suddenly too short but your chest stays narrow. Some boys get long arms before they fill out. Others notice their heads look a bit bigger or their jaw starts to change shape. It can be awkward looking at yourself and feeling out of proportion, especially when you compare yourself to friends or pictures in magazines or on TV.

Real stories help make this less scary. I once talked to a boy named Marco, who had huge feet by age twelve. He hated gym class because he felt like everyone was staring at his shoes. But by eighth grade, his height shot up, and his feet looked just right again. Another boy, Luis, had long, skinny arms that made him feel clumsy in art class. He was sure he'd never look "normal." Eventually, his muscles filled out, and he laughed, remembering how worried he'd been. Even boys from different backgrounds go through this in their own way—a friend from Korea told me his family teased him about his "noodle arms" until his shoulders broadened in high school.

These lopsided moments don't last forever. Bodies all have a plan, even if it feels random. If you're worried about being different, remember: every boy you know has something about himself that feels weird or out of sync at some point. You might not hear it in the locker room or see it on Instagram, but it's true. Even the kid who looks "perfect" probably has days where he thinks his ears stick out or his neck is too long.

The best thing you can do when you feel out-of-step is to focus on what your body can do instead of just how it looks. Maybe those big hands help you catch a baseball better or make it easier to play piano or video games. Long arms might mean you can swim faster or reach the top shelf without a stool. Even if you don't feel "in proportion" right now, your body is working hard behind the scenes to even things out.

Try not to compare yourself to friends or those "model" pictures you see everywhere. Those images are often edited or staged and don't show real growth patterns anyway. And friends who tease? Most of the time, they're just calling you out to hide their own worries about how their bodies are changing.

If you ever get stuck thinking you're not growing the "right" way, talk to someone you trust—a parent, grandparent, or even a sports coach. Most adults remember feeling out-of-place at some point. They'll tell you those feelings pass as your body keeps building itself up.

Remind yourself: it's all part of the process. No one gets everything at once; you're just leveling up in stages. You'll notice things will start to feel more balanced over time—even if it feels like forever right now.

When self-doubt creeps in, remind yourself of what your body can do today—maybe you ran faster than last week or finished your project early. Write down three things your body helped you do this week that made you proud. Being patient with yourself is huge right now.

So next time you look in the mirror and spot long toes or big hands, remember: that's just one stage of building the full "you." Give yourself some credit for making it through the awkward parts—and know that everyone else is patching together their own upgrade, too, one piece at a time.

REAL BODIES, REAL DIFFERENCES—NO ONE LOOKS LIKE THE BROCHURE

Walk down any school hallway, and you'll notice what posters and textbooks miss: real boys rarely look like the "perfect" magazine photos. Everybody grows their own way—some boys are short, others tall, some have round faces or sharp jaws, curly or straight hair, freckles, dimples, wide noses, or thin lips. Skin can be any shade, and hair grows differently for everyone. One boy might have thick eyebrows, another a patchy beard, another no chest hair yet. Seeing a group of neighborhood boys or my grandson's friends always reminds me—that there's no "right" way to look.

I've spoken to dozens of boys who've felt out of place. Samir was embarrassed by a birthmark until a friend called it cool. Jalen wished for lighter skin until he saw athletes on TV who helped him feel proud of his own. Luis wanted his freckles gone—until his younger sister tried to draw some on herself. All these boys grew up seeing different bodies at home, school, or on teams, and learned that fitting in isn't about matching, but about embracing what makes you stand out.

Textbooks and nurse's office posters usually show just one kind of body: straight posture, flawless skin, just one or two skin colors. But real life isn't like that. In gym, you'll see skinny legs next to strong thighs; one boy with big feet stands by another with tiny toes. Some boys have scars, birthmarks, or patches of dry skin. These are real, growing bodies. Not a single one matches the "brochure," and that's something to celebrate.

There's a myth about an "ideal" look—a perfect mix of height, muscles, skin color, and even how you walk. Most pictures online or in ads are edited, filtered, and staged to show just one version of "boy." No one looks like that all the time. When someone on Instagram seems flawless, remember: it likely took many tries to get that photo shoot to look perfect. Even famous athletes and actors have pimples and bad hair days.

What makes your body awesome is what makes it yours. If you're not sure what makes your body unique, look in the mirror—find your smile, dimples, the shape of your eyebrows, or the way your eyes crinkle. Your difference is your strength in believing in yourself.

Journal Prompt: What's One Thing That Makes Your Body Different and Awesome?

Write down one thing about your body that makes you proud—no matter how small. Did you carry a friend piggyback? Or maybe your freckles make a unique pattern.

Negative self-talk happens to everyone. If you catch yourself wishing you looked like someone else or thinking you're not "enough," remember: those thoughts aren't facts. If someone teases you about how you look, their words say more about them than about you. Stand tall (even if you're nervous) and reply simply: "I like my hair this way," or "Everyone grows at their own pace." Or joke: "Guess my ears are ahead of schedule." Most bullies stop when they see you're not embarrassed.

Here's a list of affirmations for tough days:

- My body is strong and lets me do what I love.
- I am proud of my differences.
- No one else looks exactly like me—and that's cool.
- My worth isn't measured by my size or shape.
- I can stand up for myself and others.

To wrap up, there's no single way to look or be a boy. Every face tells its own story. Your body is yours, growing in its own way and time, and deserves kindness and respect—especially from you. Next, we'll talk about how to keep your awesome body healthy and feeling good, because self-care is for everyone.

3

HYGIENE HEROES—MASTERING THE BASICS WITHOUT THE LECTURE

BO AND THE PITS—WHY YOU SMELL DIFFERENT AND WHAT TO DO

Have you ever found yourself in gym class suddenly wary of a strange smell—and realized it might be you? Catching a whiff of "eau de armpit" for the first time can make you feel like you've joined a secret club no one talks about. Maybe after basketball practice you get self-conscious, worrying teammates can smell you coming. The truth is that body odor (BO) sneaks up on everyone during puberty, and it can make even the most confident kid uneasy. But you're not alone, and nothing's wrong with you—your body is just upgrading, like a phone getting new features, only this time it's all about sweat and smell.

Before puberty, sweat is mostly water and salt. You could run around all day and just come home sticky, not stinky. Then, hormones activate new sweat glands, called apocrine glands, primarily located under your arms and around your groin. These glands suddenly start producing a thicker sweat full of proteins and fats. Bacteria on your skin feed on this new sweat and leave behind the familiar body odor (BO) smell.

This is different from the old sweat you got just from playing outside. Puberty sweat hangs around longer, gets trapped by new body hair, and gives bacteria more time to work their magic. That's why you might notice a strong, sometimes sour or oniony smell after gym class or on hot days. Some boys only notice it after sports, while others notice it more frequently.

It's easy to feel embarrassed or worry what friends will say, especially in gym class. You might see some guys using tons of body spray or cracking jokes about who smells "like a foot." For example, Lucas nearly skipped sleepovers, afraid friends would notice his post-basketball BO. He tried layering T-shirts, hoping to trap the smell, but only ended up sweating more. Once he asked his dad for help, he learned some tricks to take control.

There's pressure to always smell fresh, thanks to ads for "cool guy" deodorants. But you aren't alone, and you don't need to be embarrassed. Every boy goes through this. Even the kid who seems to always smell just-washed has days when his pits rebel.

What works best? Simple routines to keep you confident, even on the sweatiest days.

BO Busters—What to Do Every Day

- **Wash up:** Clean your armpits with soap and warm water each morning and after sports.
- **Dry off:** Bacteria thrive on damp skin; dry your armpits before getting dressed.
- **Change clothes:** Put on fresh shirts, socks, and underwear daily.

HYGIENE HEROES—MASTERING THE BASICS WITHOUT THE... | 45

- **Choose breathable fabrics:** Cotton helps sweat dry and prevents trapping odors.
- **Pack extras:** Keep an extra shirt in your locker or bag for after gym.
- **Ask for help:** Talk to someone at home or school if you're worried about BO.

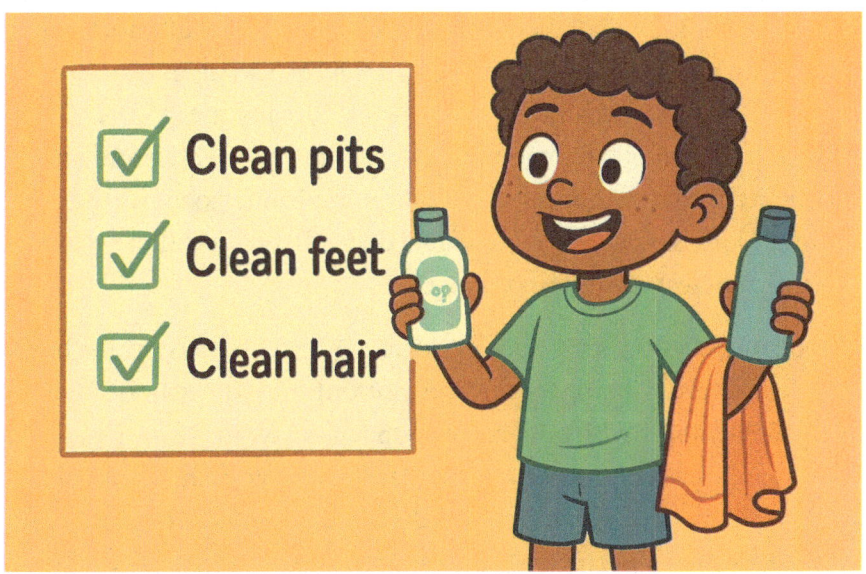

If someone comments on your BO ("Whoa, someone smells!"), don't panic. You can lighten it with humor ("Guess my superpower's working overtime!") or just say, "Thanks for letting me know." Everyone deals with this sooner or later.

It's also okay to talk about it at home. You can say, "Hey, I think I need help with BO," or "Can we get some stuff for my pits?" Most parents have been there and are glad you brought it up.

Managing BO is really about comfort and not letting it get in the way of school or fun. With a few easy steps, you can focus on what really matters without stressing out every time you lift your arms.

Puberty brings new changes, but learning to handle BO helps you stay confident and in control every day.

DEODORANT DECODER—HOW, WHEN, AND WHY TO START USING IT

You've probably seen those colorful sticks and sprays in stores promising things like "Ocean Blast" or "Extreme Sport," and maybe you've watched older family members use them. Deodorant isn't some mysterious adult secret—it's for anyone whose sweat has started to smell stronger, thanks to puberty. Deodorant covers up or neutralizes odor, while antiperspirant goes further by helping block sweat. Some products do both, but you don't need to pick the fanciest option on the shelf.

When should you start? There's no set age. Some boys notice body odor as early as nine or ten; others not until middle school. If your pits smell sour or strong after gym class, that's your signal. It doesn't matter when your friends start—everyone hits this phase at their own pace. If you need deodorant before or after your classmates, that's perfectly fine. As one reader, Tyler, asked, "What if I'm the only one in my class using deodorant?" The answer: it's about your body's needs, not everyone else's schedule. Feeling fresh and confident is always the right call.

Shopping for deodorant doesn't need to be a big production, though the wall of choices can feel overwhelming. For support, bring a parent or older sibling. Check the labels: some say "deodorant," some "antiperspirant," and others are combos. If you have sensitive skin, look for "unscented" or "for sensitive skin." Stronger scents are fine, but milder is safer if you're worried about clashing with cologne or body spray. There are also natural options that are free from aluminum and artificial fragrances, which are worth trying if your skin is sensitive.

A simple first deodorant shopping list:

- Deodorant stick (unscented or lightly scented)
- Antiperspirant (for heavy sweaters)
- Sensitive skin formula (if you get rashes)
- Travel-sized stick (for the gym or sleepovers)

Don't stress about picking what everyone else has. Start with something mild, and see how your skin reacts after a few days.

Applying deodorant for the first time is easy. Make sure your pits are clean and dry—don't put it on sweaty skin right after gym. Hold the stick or roll-on at the bottom, twist up a little, and swipe under each arm three or four times for full coverage without excess. For sprays, hold six inches from your skin and quickly spray under each arm. Cap it when done, and wash your hands if there's any residue.

Deodorant Dos and Don'ts

Do:

- Use deodorant daily after showering.
- Choose a formula comfortable for your skin.
- Try different brands if one irritates you.
- Ask for help if you're unsure.

Don't:

- Share deodorant (it spreads germs).
- Overdo it—a little goes a long way.
- Apply to broken or irritated skin.
- Forget to check for white marks on shirts before leaving.

If you forget deodorant and worry at school or practice, relax—most people are too busy to notice unless you call attention to it. If anyone asks or teases you about using deodorant early, shrug and reply, "I like to smell good,"—then move on.

If deodorant irritates your skin or causes bumps, consider switching brands or trying unscented options. If you get a persistent rash, tell an adult so they can help find something safe for you.

There's nothing embarrassing about when you start using deodorant. It simply means your body is changing. Choose whatever makes you feel comfortable and confident. Next time you see those bright, colorful deodorants in the store, remember: they're just tools for feeling good in your own skin.

SHOWER POWER—MAKING BATHING EASY (EVEN ON LAZY DAYS)

Showering during puberty is a whole new game. Your body is busy building muscle, growing taller, and working overtime, which means you sweat more than you did as a little kid. Sports, gym class, running around at recess, or even just sitting in a warm classroom can leave you feeling sticky or smelly. Even if you can't see the sweat, your skin is working hard every day. You might feel like skipping a shower sometimes. Maybe you're tired or you think, "I barely did anything today." But the truth is, showers matter more than ever now. Skipping just one can turn your "fresh" feeling into "funky" in no time. There's also the science of sweat to think about.

Sweat itself doesn't really smell bad; it's the bacteria on your skin that throws the stink party. When sweat sits on skin, bacteria breaks it down to make that classic "locker room" smell. Washing

HYGIENE HEROES—MASTERING THE BASICS WITHOUT THE... | 49

away both sweat and bacteria keeps you fresher for longer, even after tough practices.

A shower isn't just about standing underwater for five seconds and calling it done. There's a right way to get clean and ensure you don't miss those trouble spots that can become ripe quickly.

Start with warm water—not too hot or cold—so you're comfortable. Use a gentle soap or body wash and lather up your whole body.

Pay extra attention to your armpits, groin area, feet, and the back of your ears. These spots trap sweat and oil, and can be easy to miss if you rush.

Take time to wash between your toes and the back of your neck—those are sneaky places for grime to hide. Rinse off thoroughly so no soap residue is left behind, which can cause itchy skin. **Using a washcloth** or loofah helps scrub away dead skin. After rinsing, dry off completely with a clean towel before getting dressed so bacteria don't get a head start.

Shower Checklist

- Start with warm water.
- Use enough soap to lather up.
- Wash your armpits well.
- Clean around your groin and between your legs.
- Scrub your feet, especially between the toes.
- Wash behind ears and neck.
- Rinse off all soap.
- Dry off fully before getting dressed.

Some days you'll hear yourself say, "I don't have time," or "I'll do it tomorrow." Maybe you forget because you get distracted by video games or homework. Sometimes, you might just not feel like it. If this sounds familiar, there are ways to make showers quicker and more fun so they're less of a chore and more of a reward for making it through the day. Try showering at the same time every morning or night to build a habit—right after waking up or before bed works for most guys. For super busy mornings, keep your shower to five minutes: soap up, scrub, rinse, done. If you know you have practice or PE tomorrow, plan to shower right after. Set reminders on your phone or leave sticky notes in the bathroom if forgetting is a problem.

Turning shower time into self-care is way better than treating it like punishment. Crank up your favorite playlist, or grab a waterproof speaker if you want music. Make up goofy songs about scrubbing your feet or time yourself and see if you can beat yesterday's record for "quickest clean." Give yourself silly rewards—like picking tomorrow's breakfast—if you stick to your shower routine all week. If you finish strong after a hard day or tough practice, picture washing away all the stress with the sweat.

Everyone likes feeling fresh and clean—even if no one else says it out loud. You'll notice you walk taller when you know you don't stink, and classmates notice, too (but in a good way). Getting clean isn't just about stopping BO; it's about resetting after long days, cooling down after being nervous before a test, or warming up after playing outside in the cold.

Shower objections come up all the time, but there's usually a fix that works for everyone. If you hate being cold, pick a warmer part of the day or use a fluffy towel straight from the dryer. For those who rush because they're bored, try bringing in a toy basketball hoop or timing your shampoo rinse with the beat of a favorite song. If water feels weird on your skin, try standing near the edge at first and working up to longer showers.

HYGIENE HEROES—MASTERING THE BASICS WITHOUT THE ... | 51

Here's something to celebrate:

- Every time you shower without being nagged? *Achievement unlocked!*
- Survived Monday after soccer? *Achievement unlocked!*
- Washed behind both ears for the first time ever? *Achievement unlocked!*

Make your own list of **"Shower Wins"** and see how many badges you can collect in a week.

Showering thoroughly keeps skin healthy, helps prevent breakouts, and makes you feel ready for whatever comes next at school, practice, or home. Plus, nothing beats the feeling of slipping into clean clothes when you're squeaky clean underneath.

CLOTHES, SOCKS, AND UNDERWEAR—HOW OFTEN TO CHANGE & WHY IT MATTERS

Pulling on fresh socks or clean underwear might sound like no big deal, but it's one of the biggest game-changers for feeling comfortable and confident each day. When you start to sweat more during puberty, your clothes soak up that sweat right along with you. Old sweat plus bacteria equals a recipe for stinky shirts, socks that could knock out a rhino, and underwear you seriously would not want anyone to see. Changing these clothes daily—or even more often if you're playing sports or running around a lot—doesn't just keep you smelling good. It helps your skin stay healthy, prevents itchy rashes, and stops bacteria from turning tiny problems into bigger ones. You might not notice right away, but skipping too many changes can lead to red patches, itchy skin, or even an infection. Have you ever had a day when you kept the same socks on after gym class, and then your feet started itching like crazy?

That's a sign the sweat and bacteria are having a party they shouldn't be having.

Wearing the same underwear or socks for days in a row can also lead to some seriously embarrassing moments. There's the story of Cameron, who wore his favorite soccer socks all week because he didn't want to bother with laundry. By Friday, his feet were so smelly that his friends started calling him "Stink Bomb." He laughed it off, but inside, he felt embarrassed and wished he'd just grabbed a clean pair. The same goes for underwear—a quick change in the morning can save you from itching, chafing, or unwanted attention in the locker room. Sometimes life gets busy, laundry piles up, or you just forget. But it's always easier to fix it early than try to ignore it.

One of the secrets to always having something clean is getting into a routine that works for you. Some people like to lay out tomorrow's clothes before bed: shirt, pants, socks, and underwear all ready to go, so there's no guesswork in the morning. Others set reminders on their phone or use sticky notes on their dresser as a nudge. If you play sports or have gym at school, try packing extra socks and underwear in your bag. That way, you can change right after practice and feel fresh for the rest of the day. Tying new habits to things you already do helps, too—change into clean socks right after brushing your teeth or swap out underwear before breakfast. The more automatic it feels, the less likely you'll forget.

Running out of clean clothes happens to everyone sooner or later. You might dig through your drawer and realize there are no clean shirts left, or only have one sock that matches. Sometimes, it's embarrassing to ask for help—maybe you don't want to admit you forgot, or you worry someone will be annoyed. But parents and caregivers know laundry is part of growing up. If you're stuck, try saying something simple like, "Hey, I ran out of clean socks—can

HYGIENE HEROES—MASTERING THE BASICS WITHOUT THE... | 53

we do laundry tonight?" or "I need help learning how to wash my clothes." Most adults would rather help than see you struggle.

How To Do Laundry

Start by sorting dirty clothes—keep underwear and socks together with shirts and pants in a separate pile. Use cold water if you're not sure; it works for most things and won't shrink your favorite hoodie. Add detergent (ask someone at home how much if you're new at this), then hit start and wait for the magic to happen. When the wash is done, move everything to the dryer or hang it up if needed. Folding isn't fun, but it keeps things from getting wrinkled and smelly again. Learning to do laundry yourself is a win for everyone.

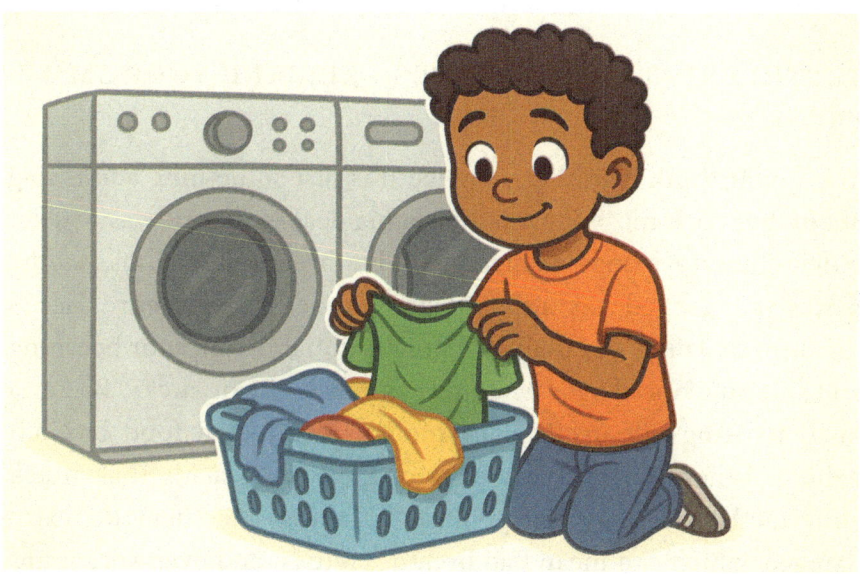

If you forget how to do any step, there's no shame in asking for a quick refresher or checking an online video together with someone at home. The main thing is not being afraid to speak up about laundry needs—nobody expects you to know everything right away.

Changing clothes daily is about more than just avoiding funny looks at school or sidestepping locker room jokes. It helps your skin breathe, stops bacteria from building up, and gives you a boost of confidence every single day. Clean clothes also mean a lower chance of breakouts around your waistline, thighs, or feet—places where sweat tends to hide. If your skin starts feeling itchy under your waistband or your feet get red between the toes, that's your body asking for a fresh start.

Forgetting to change now and then happens to everyone. Just do your best to make it part of your daily routine and ask for help if laundry ever feels overwhelming. You'll be surprised how much better you feel heading into your day with something fresh on top and bottom—even if nobody else notices but you.

TEETH, BREATH, AND BRACES—KEEPING YOUR SMILE FRESH

You might think brushing your teeth is just something adults nag about, but trust me, your mouth is a big deal—especially as you get older. Puberty brings changes to your breath and gums, so the basics you learned as a little kid start to matter even more. Here's the deal: morning and night are non-negotiable times for brushing and skipping one. That's when things get smelly or sticky. Bacteria loves to hang out inside your mouth, feeding on food bits left behind. When they party too hard, they make acids that attack your teeth and gums. Skipping a brushing lets them do extra damage, which can mean bad breath, cavities, and even sore gums that bleed when you floss. None of those are fun at all.

If you ever wonder why your breath suddenly seems stronger or "funky," you're not alone. Hormones change how much you drool (saliva production) and how your gums react to plaque. Add in eating more snacks, maybe sleeping with your mouth open, or

HYGIENE HEROES—MASTERING THE BASICS WITHOUT THE... | 55

going through a phase where you like spicy food, and your breath can go from "okay" to "whoa" pretty fast. The best way to fight back is simple: brush with fluoride toothpaste for two full minutes every morning and night. Don't just swipe the front—get the backs of your teeth, the gumline, and your tongue, too. That's where most of the bacteria hides out.

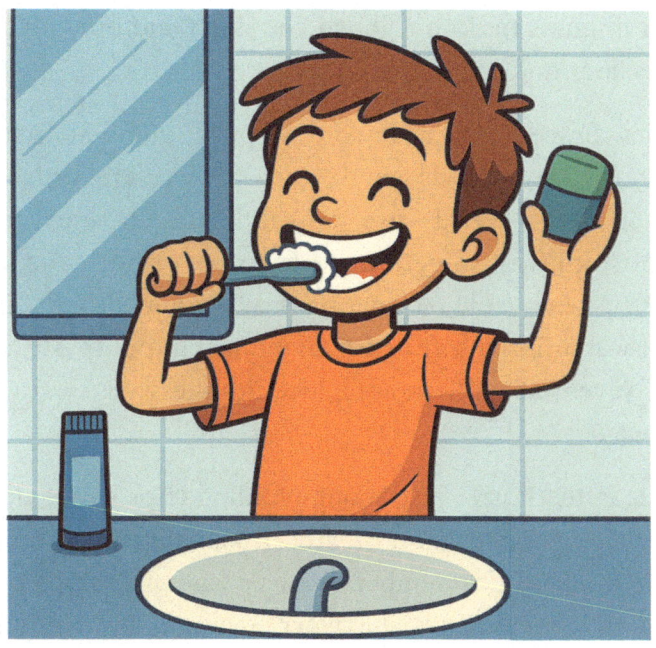

Flossing seems like an annoying step, but it's what gets the gunk from between your teeth that your brush misses. If you skip flossing, you're leaving behind a buffet for bacteria. Floss once a day, wiggling gently between each tooth. If regular floss feels tricky, try those plastic floss picks—they make it easier to reach the back. Mouthwash helps knock out extra germs and gives your breath a bonus boost. If mouthwash feels too strong, use water or chew sugar-free gum after eating. Drinking water during the day also helps wash away food bits and keeps your mouth from getting dry (which makes your breath worse).

Braces bring their own set of challenges—suddenly, there are brackets and wires that trap food in places you never noticed before. If you have braces, brushing after every meal is the best way to keep stuff from sticking around and causing odors or stains. Use a soft brush and take time around each bracket. Special tools like floss threaders or small "tree-shaped" brushes get under the wires where normal brushes can't reach. It's worth taking a few extra minutes to do it right so you don't end up with stains or sore spots later on.

Sometimes, braces can cause sore or puffy gums at first. That's normal, but it still needs gentle care. Don't skip brushing just because it feels weird—use a gentle touch and let your orthodontist know if something feels wrong or hurts for too long. If you have a removable retainer or clear aligner, clean it every day with cool water and a soft brush (avoid using toothpaste, as it can scratch). Never eat with an appliance in unless your orthodontist says it's okay.

Having clean teeth isn't just about avoiding trips to the dentist or getting yelled at for "dragon breath." It actually changes how you feel about yourself. I remember one boy who almost never smiled in school pictures because he worried about his teeth looking yellow or his breath being bad around friends. Once he started brushing better and using mouthwash every day, he felt more confident and smiling more in class, talking to new people, and even answering questions out loud without worrying someone would notice something off with his breath. Clean teeth make you feel sharp, prepared, and ready for whatever comes up at school or anywhere else.

If you want to make dentist visits easier (and trust me, everyone does), keep track of how often you brush and floss each week. Mark it on a calendar or use an app if that's easier for you. Every time you check off both morning and night brushing, give yourself a little credit—those small wins add up fast.

Besides feeling fresher, taking care of your mouth gives great first impressions—whether you're meeting a new teacher, hanging with friends after school, or talking to someone special for the first time. No one wants to worry about hiding their smile or covering their mouth when they laugh.

Regular brushing and flossing might sound boring compared to all the other stuff happening in puberty, but they set you up for fewer problems later. And honestly? There's no feeling better than waking up with fresh breath and knowing your smile is ready for anything.

As you keep building these healthy habits—washing up, keeping clothes clean, caring for skin—don't forget your teeth are part of the whole package, too. A fresh mouth makes every day feel brighter and opens doors to new connections at school, sports, and everywhere else.

So now that you've got your hygiene game strong from head to toe (and everywhere in between), get set for what comes next: figuring out emotions, mood swings, and all the stuff happening inside your mind as well as outside. That's up next—and trust me, it matters just as much as keeping clean does.

4

BRAINWAVES & MOOD SWINGS— YOUR CHANGING MIND AND EMOTIONS

MOOD SWINGS: WHY YOU SOMETIMES SNAP (AND HOW TO CHILL OUT)

Imagine you're playing a game with your brother, he nudges you by accident, and suddenly you're yelling or stomping off as if he ruined everything. Minutes later, you feel bad, puzzled, or you might even laugh at yourself for overreacting. Or perhaps you're laughing with friends and, out of nowhere, get annoyed and want to be alone. If this sounds familiar, you're not alone. This is classic puberty brain at work.

During puberty, your brain gets a major "software update." Think of your brain as a phone that's suddenly downloading new, mysterious apps—these apps are hormones. Hormones like testosterone spread throughout your body, prompting rapid changes. Your emotions bounce around more than ever. You may snap, laugh, cry, or get annoyed—all within an hour. It doesn't mean something's wrong with you; your brain is simply learning some new tricks.

Science Facts

There's real science behind these mood swings. The prefrontal cortex—the part responsible for thinking things through and controlling impulses—is still developing. Meanwhile, the amygdala, the emotional center, is running the show. That's why emotions can take over before your logical brain even catches up. It's like putting a powerful engine into a fragile frame: lots of power, not much control. So small things (like someone taking the last cookie or your phone dying) can hit your nerves harder than they might have before. Remember, all adults went through this too, and some are still figuring it out.

Why Am I Sad or Angry for No Reason? —Understanding New Emotions

Mood swings show up in everyday situations. You might get irritated by a simple question at dinner, feel picked on after a harmless joke, or go from cheerful at breakfast to moody by lunch for no particular reason. It isn't just anger—you might be laughing at a meme one moment, then suddenly want to be left alone. These emotions come and go quickly. Sometimes, you might slam a door or say things you don't mean, only to regret it later or wonder why you felt so strongly.

Talking about emotions can be tough, especially when you don't understand them yourself. Often, you say you're "fine" when you want to hide in your room or shout into a pillow. To help, try breaking emotions into smaller parts. Imagine feelings as colors on a wheel, each with a name—not just happy or sad. You might be frustrated (when homework is hard), embarrassed (when someone notices your new haircut), nervous (before a game), excited (after a popular post), or bored (waiting for the weekend). Naming your feelings can make them less scary and help clarify your mood—a feeling, not a permanent state.

You aren't broken and you are definitely not alone, absolutely everyone experiences mood swings during puberty. Some people just hide them better. Adults all have stories about snapping at their parents or getting mad over nothing when they were your age. It's comforting to remember this is totally normal; it's just your brain growing and learning to handle bigger feelings and decisions.

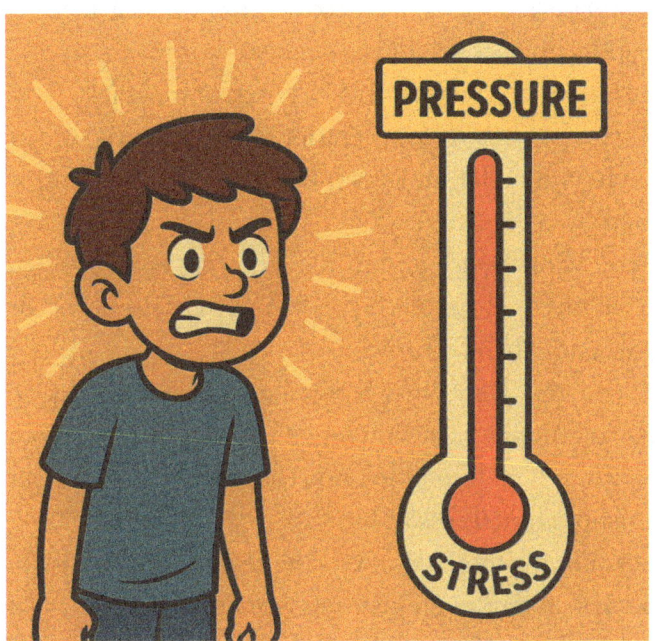

Talking About Emotions Can be Tough Q & A

Q. So, what can you do when you feel like you're about to snap?

Try these answers, maybe one will work for you this time and another one next time...

- A. Try to notice the early warning signs: maybe your fists clench, your heart races, or your face gets hot. These are signs it's time to pause.
- A. One quick way to calm down is "box breathing": breathe in for four seconds, hold it for four seconds, breathe out for four seconds, then hold again for four seconds. Picture drawing a box as you count. Do this three times and you might start to relax.
- A. If counting isn't your style, try stepping away for a minute. Say, "I need a quick break," and move to another room, go outside, or splash cold water on your face.
- A. If your muscles are tense, squeeze a pillow, a stress ball, or even a rolled-up sock until the tension passes.
- A. Music helps many people too. Make a playlist of songs that help you chill out. Listen with headphones until you feel better.
- A. If you want, pause and think: What three words describe how you feel? Maybe "calm, tired, hopeful" or "annoyed, confused, bored."
- A. Or you can draw your mood—just sketch shapes or colors that match how you feel. One boy drew a storm cloud when he felt mad for no reason; another made a tiny dot to show loneliness at lunch.
- A. Journaling helps, too, if talking feels hard. Write how you feel each day, even just one word like "blank," "okay," or "over it." Even "I don't know" is a good start.

Over time, you might notice patterns—maybe you're always grumpy after school on Mondays or tired before big tests. Recognizing these patterns helps you understand yourself better.

Putting your mood on paper or naming it often makes things feel lighter and less overwhelming. You might realize being sad or mad isn't as big as it felt inside.

Mood Swing Buster: Your Quick Reset Checklist

- Spot your warning signs (clenched hands, fast heartbeat)
- Try box breathing: In 4 sec, Hold 4, Out 4, Hold 4 (repeat three times)
- Step away for some fresh air
- Squeeze a pillow or stress ball
- Listen to your 'chill' playlist to help reset
- 3- words list
- Draw your mood, sketch how you feel
- Journal

It takes some practice to notice and manage mood swings before they blow up. Every time you calm yourself—even a little—you're building valuable life skills that many adults wish they had mastered. Mood swings are a normal part of growing up, but learning to handle them really sets you apart.

Some days, everything goes right—you laugh with friends, win a game, eat your favorite lunch—yet, suddenly, you feel sad or irritated for no clear reason. You may wonder if something's wrong or if you're alone in feeling this way. For example, one of my boys once had a great day at school but came home quiet and down. When asked, he simply said, "I don't know. I just feel weird." This stuck with me, as so many boys experience these unexplained feelings. You don't always need a reason—sometimes, emotions just happen without warning.

Puberty can flip a switch on your emotions. Where you once felt happy, mad, or a little upset, now you might experience frustration when your phone acts up, embarrassment because of a comment, nervousness before a game, or sudden excitement that turns to anxiety. These emotions can feel intense—making your chest tight or your stomach clench—or, at times, you might feel nothing at all and wonder why things don't interest you anymore. These changes are your brain growing and making new connections. You aren't broken, and you're definitely not alone.

When big emotions surprise you, remember that no feeling is forever. Even the strongest moods will shift over time, though it may not feel like it right away. If a feeling gets too strong and disrupts your day, try moving around, talking to someone you trust, or doing something creative—building, gaming, or drawing.

Others experience similar emotions—friends, siblings, teachers, parents. That friend who snaps at lunch might be dealing with his own tough feelings. Everyone has days when they can't explain their mood.

Growing up is about meeting these emotions as they come—even when they don't make sense. Learning to notice and name your feelings is a key skill. Most importantly, it reminds you that feeling weird sometimes is one of the most normal parts of growing up.

REAL TALK: WHEN YOU WANT TO BE ALONE (IT'S OKAY)

Sometimes, an odd feeling creeps in—you get foggy, everything's noisy, and you just want to shut your door and be alone. You might feel this way at family dinners, with friends, or in class, wishing for some space. That's normal, especially during puberty when your brain is extra busy. Wanting time alone isn't strange, rude, or a sign you're becoming a hermit. It's actually one of the best ways to recharge, kind of like plugging in your phone after a long day.

Needing space doesn't mean you dislike people. It's not about ignoring friends or family—it's just that your brain gets full sometimes. Noise, conversation, schoolwork, even fun times can pile up and leave you overwhelmed. That's called overstimulation. It often hits after busy weekends, long school days, or tough activities. Sometimes it's obvious—a noisy classroom or too many conversations. Other times it sneaks up: maybe a tough test or long practice leaves you drained and craving quiet.

People don't often talk about why time alone matters, but it helps you process your feelings and thoughts. Taking breaks lets your brain sort out the day—good, bad, or confusing—so you can reset. Alone time can make you less cranky, more focused, and even creative. Some of your best ideas might come when you're on your own.

There's a myth that wanting space is rude or weird—don't believe it. Adults need alone time too. If people ask why you're quiet or seem off, it's fine to say you need a break. Wanting space isn't about hurting others; it's just self-care.

Sometimes people misunderstand. They may think you're upset with them. To help, use simple words that explain: "I need a few minutes to myself, I'll come back soon," or "I'm not mad, just need quiet right now." These reassure others without hurting feelings.

If someone pushes for more—like a sibling who keeps talking or a parent who has questions—you can say, "Can I talk to you in a bit? I just need time alone first." Most people understand when you explain, and you don't have to go into big details. Even "I'm just tired" is usually enough.

Alone time doesn't have to be boring or lonely. It's a chance to do things that relax and recharge you: read, listen to music, draw, walk around the block, build something with LEGO, or play solo games. Choose what you like—scribbling in a notebook, sketching random stuff, or building playlists can all help. Music, especially playlists for different moods, gives comfort when things feel heavy.

If being alone ever feels too quiet or lonely, switch things up—pet your dog, organize stuff, or watch funny videos. After a little time alone, you may feel ready to be social again—or at least ready for dinner without feeling overwhelmed.

The key is to use alone time to listen to what you need. If you start to feel restless or bored, that's your signal that you've recharged enough and can handle being around people again.

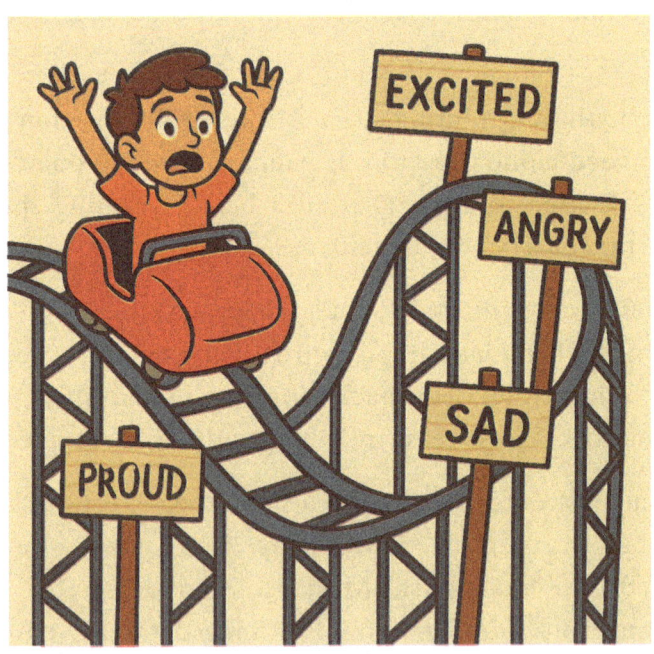

Pay attention to what triggers your need for space and what helps you recharge. Maybe noise feels worse on Mondays or crowds exhaust you after practice. When you spot patterns, you can plan ahead—bring headphones for a bus ride or keep a book handy at school.

Everyone needs different amounts of alone time, and your needs may change from week to week. Some days you'll want lots of space, other days hardly any. All of that is normal.

Learning to ask for alone time kindly—and knowing how to use it well—will help you now and long-term. You'll take care of yourself and keep your relationships strong, even if others don't always understand right away.

COPING WITH ANXIETY—SIMPLE TRICKS THAT ACTUALLY WORK

Anxiety is sneaky. It can sneak up when you least expect it, making your heart race or your stomach feel like you swallowed a handful of butterflies. Sometimes it shows up as sweaty palms, shaky knees, or a mind that just won't stop spinning. You might sit in class and suddenly worry everyone is looking at you. Or you might stare at a blank test and feel your brain freeze like a computer that won't load. Anxiety is like getting stuck in a loop where your thoughts run wild and your body follows along for the ride. This feeling is common, not just for kids, but for adults too—though they try to hide it with coffee and fake smiles.

Think about all the times your brain has gone into overdrive for no real reason. You may worry before a big test, joining a new team, talking in front of the class, or even sending a text to a group chat. My oldest grandson once got so anxious before his first sleepover that he asked to pack his own snacks (just in case he got hungry), made sure his favorite pillow was ready, and then nearly backed out at the last minute because "What if I snore?" He ended up having fun and was so glad he went, but it took a lot of courage to walk through that door. Nerves can hit before school trips, church camp, at the orthodontist, or when you try something new—like speaking up for yourself or making friends with someone who seems really cool.

Anxiety rarely sticks to just one shape. Sometimes it's a ball of energy in your belly, other times it's a heavy feeling that makes you want to skip out on things. It can make your thoughts race ahead, worrying about what might happen next or what could go wrong. This is normal—your brain's natural way of trying to protect you. It doesn't always get it right, though. Most of the time, the things you worry about never even happen.

There are tricks you can use anywhere, even in the middle of class or at a crowded lunch table. One is called the "5-4-3-2-1" grounding trick. Look around and quietly name five things you see—a pencil, your shoe, the clock, a friend's backpack, the teacher's shoes. Next, touch four things—your desk, your sleeve, your chair, your pencil case. Then listen for three sounds—the hum of the lights, someone shuffling papers, someone laughing in the hallway. Next, notice two smells—the soap from your hands, maybe lunch from the cafeteria. Finally, taste one thing—even if it's just the inside of your mouth or a sip of water. This trick pulls your brain back to what's real and right in front of you, instead of letting it run--a- muck with wild stories.

Another easy trick is visualization. Close your eyes for a moment (or just stare at a spot on the floor if that feels less awkward) and picture your favorite peaceful place. Maybe it's your bedroom with soft blankets, a quiet corner in the library, or sitting on grass under a tree with sunlight on your face. Imagine every detail—what it sounds like, what it smells like, how safe it feels there. Even thirty seconds can help reset your mood and make your thoughts less jumpy.

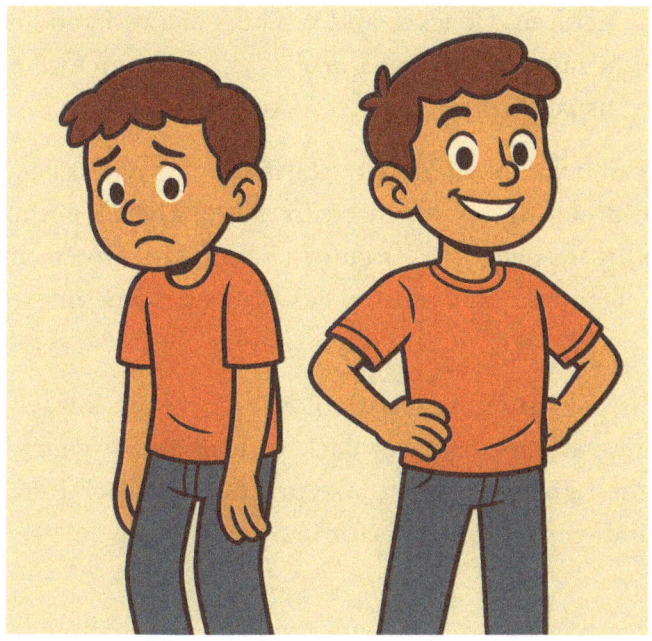

Sometimes worries feel sticky and won't leave on their own, no matter how hard you try to ignore them. When that happens, try the "worry box" idea. Grab some paper and write down whatever keeps buzzing in your head—"I'm nervous about my science project," "I don't want to mess up at soccer," "What if I forget my lines in the play?" Fold each worry and drop it into a shoebox or jar. You can even decorate it to make it yours. Tell yourself you'll deal with those worries later—after dinner, after school, or after practice—and put the box away for now. Just moving those worries out of your head and onto paper can help them feel less daunting.

If anxiety gets too big or sticks around too long, don't keep it to yourself. Even grown-ups sometimes need help with worry. Reach out to someone who makes you feel safe—maybe a parent, grandparent, or older sibling who understands. School counselors are there for this exact reason; they won't judge or make fun of you for feeling nervous. Coaches and teachers are also good choices—they've seen hundreds of kids deal with nerves before games or events and usually know some tricks to help.

Doctors can help, too, if anxiety starts to mess with sleep or stops you from doing things you used to enjoy. There's nothing weak about asking for help; it takes guts to admit when you're struggling with big feelings. Everyone needs backup sometimes—parents included.

You don't have to fight anxiety alone. There are always ways to shrink those worries and get back to feeling like yourself again. Finding the right trick might take practice, but each time you try, you're building stronger skills for life.

SELF-KINDNESS AND YOUR INNER COACH—HOW TO TALK TO YOURSELF

There's always a voice running in your head—a kind of narrator for your life. Sometimes, it cheers you on, other times it's harsh. This is your "inner voice" or self-talk. During puberty, when everything feels uncertain, that inner voice often gets louder. You'll notice it when you look in the mirror, try new things, or make mistakes. How you talk to yourself really matters: it can soften hard days or make small problems feel huge. Negative self-talk sounds like, "I'm so weird," "I'll never get this," or "Everyone else is better than me." It sneaks in until you believe it. Positive self-coaching flips those thoughts: "I'm learning," "Everyone makes mistakes," or "This will pass." The key is to notice which voice is dominant and practice letting your kinder inner coach speak up more often.

Most boys have rough thoughts after messing up. Thinking, "I'm a loser," after tripping in the hallway or, "Why am I like this?" when you say something awkward is normal. But these thoughts act like bullies in your brain. You can kick them out by changing your words. Here's a quick guide:

Instead of this...Try this... "I always mess up." "Mistakes help me learn." "Nobody likes me." "Some people get me, some don't." "I'm so weird." "Everyone feels awkward sometimes." "I'll never get better at this." "I can improve if I keep going." "Why bother?" "It's worth trying again."

Say you drop your tray in the cafeteria. Your first thought is probably, "I'm such a disaster." Instead, try, "Everyone messes up sometimes," or "That was embarrassing, but it happens to everyone." These words won't erase what happened, but they help you feel less alone and more able to move on.

Practicing self-kindness takes effort, especially after mistakes. Try talking to yourself as you would talk to a friend. If your friend bombed a quiz, you wouldn't say, "You're hopeless." You'd say, "You'll get it next time." You deserve that same kindness. If you catch yourself thinking something harsh, pause and ask, "Would I say this to someone else?" If the answer is no, change your thought.

It can help to write down kind messages and keep them somewhere you'll see them—on your phone, a sticky note in your backpack, or inside your locker. When your negative voice pipes up, read one of your notes. The more you repeat these, the more natural it gets.

Try these simple affirmations or mantras when things feel rough:

Affirmation Reminders

- "I can handle this."
- "I'm not alone in how I feel."
- "I am growing and that's awesome."
- "One mistake doesn't define me."
- "I learn something new every day."
- "My feelings are real and they matter."

Pick one or make your own—short and true for you is what counts.

If being kind to yourself feels awkward or fake, that's normal. Most people think they have to be tough all the time. But self-kindness isn't about ignoring your problems or pretending things are fine. It's about letting yourself be human: to stumble, try again, and still believe you matter.

Here's something you can do: Whenever you catch a negative thought, say it out loud if you can, then answer it with a helpful message—even if you don't quite believe it yet.

For example:

Thought: "I'm so awkward."
Reply: "Everyone feels awkward sometimes. It won't last forever."

Or:

Thought: "I can't do this."
Reply: "This is hard now, but I'll get better."

The more often you practice swapping out negative thoughts for supportive ones, the easier it becomes to coach yourself instead of criticizing.

Your inner voice is yours to train. It might start off sounding strict or mean, but it doesn't have to stay that way. Over time, you can make it sound like your favorite coach or a supportive friend. Each time you do, you build confidence and strength that will last far beyond puberty.

GROWTH MINDSET: BUILDING RESILIENCE AFTER A TOUGH DAY

Some days just feel rough. Maybe you tried out for a new team, missed every goal, and walked home thinking you'd never get better. Or you studied hard for a quiz only to see a grade that made your stomach drop. It's easy to believe these moments mean you aren't good enough or that you're just not cut out for certain things. But what if you could see setbacks as part of getting better, not proof that you're stuck? That's what a "growth mindset" is all about—believing you can improve with effort, practice, and time.

Take the story of Josh. He joined the basketball team because his friends did, but at first he couldn't dribble without losing the ball. His layups bounced off the rim more times than he could count. Every practice felt like proof he didn't belong. A few weeks in, Josh wanted to quit. His coach encouraged him, though, saying, "Nobody starts as a pro. The ones who improve are the ones who keep trying." So Josh kept showing up. He watched teammates, asked for tips, and practiced at home while his dog watched. Slowly, his dribble got smoother, and he made his first basket during a scrimmage. Josh realized that each miss was teaching his muscles and brain what to do next time. By the end of the season, he was still not the best player, but he was a lot better than day one —and way more confident.

A fixed mindset sounds like,

"I'm just bad at this," or "I'll never get it right." It makes you feel stuck, as if ability is something you either have or don't have.

For example, someone with a fixed mindset after failing a math test might say, "I'm bad at math."

A growth mindset says,

I can learn this if I put in the effort," or "Mistakes help me get better." It's about seeing your brain like a muscle—each time you try something hard, it gets stronger.

Someone with a growth mindset would say, "This was tough, but I can improve if I keep practicing and ask for help."

When you've had a tough day and it feels like nothing went right, there are steps you can take to bounce back instead of giving up. First, look for what went okay, even if it's small. Maybe you remembered your gym clothes or helped someone pick up their books after class. Write down three things that didn't go horribly, no matter how minor they seem. This helps your brain spot progress and not just problems. If something was especially rough, talk about it with someone you trust—maybe a parent, grandparent, coach, or friend. Sometimes saying things out loud makes them less scary and helps you see what you can do differently next time.

It's also helpful to reframe what happened. Instead of thinking, "That presentation was a disaster," try thinking, "I did my best today and now I know what to practice." If you feel stuck on a mistake, remember it's just one moment, not your whole story.

You can always ask for help or advice. Most people love sharing tips because they've been there too.

Setting small goals is another way to build resilience. Try making your goals simple and realistic—like "I'll practice dribbling for ten minutes," or "I'll ask one question in class tomorrow." When you reach even tiny goals, celebrate that win. Keep track in a "small wins" journal or use stickers as progress badges in your notebook or on your calendar. Seeing those badges build up reminds you that every step counts.

You don't have to be perfect to be proud of yourself. Progress is about moving forward, even if it's slow. If something takes longer than you hoped, that's okay. Learning is not a race.

As this chapter wraps up, keep in mind that growing up is more about learning from challenges than avoiding them. Your mind is flexible—ready to learn new things every day if you let it. Next up: friendships, squads, and figuring out where you fit as things around you keep changing. You're not alone in this; there's always room to grow.

HI THERE, AMAZING READER!

Are you enjoying *The Essential Boy's Guide to Puberty & Body Changes, Ages 8-14* so far? Your feedback means the world to me and helps other readers discover this book.

If you're finding the content helpful, inspiring, or just plain fun, I'd be incredibly grateful if you could take a moment to share your thoughts in an Amazon review. It doesn't have to be long—just a few sentences about what you like most would make a big difference!

Scan the QR code to leave a review.

Thank you for being part of this journey and for supporting my work. Happy reading!

Warmly,

- DebbieAnn

5

SQUAD GOALS—FRIENDSHIPS, TEASING, AND SOCIAL SUPERPOWERS

BUILDING YOUR SQUAD—FINDING FRIENDS WHO GET YOU

You know that feeling when you walk into a room and see a group laughing about something you don't get? Or overhear kids chatting about a game or show you barely know? Sometimes it feels like everyone else has their squad, and you're just hoping not to eat lunch alone. Finding real friends isn't always easy, especially as you grow or your interests change. Many boys worry about being cool enough or having enough friends, but what really matters is finding people who "get" and accept you—those who make you comfortable being yourself, even on your weird days.

So, what matters in a friend? It's not about popularity or fancy sneakers. Real friends show respect, treat you well even when no one's watching, remember what you like, and include you in conversations and games. A true friend won't mock your interests—they listen and ask questions. Good friends stand up for each other and share jokes that don't hurt anyone. If someone's only around when it's convenient or when you have something they want, that's not real friendship.

How do you find these people? Start with your own interests. Maybe you like building things, gaming, drawing, sports, or music. Join a club, team, or online group around those hobbies, and you'll meet others who share your passions. For example, my son once felt alone after his old friend group drifted, but joining the school robotics club introduced him to new friends who shared his excitement. Your friend group can change as your interests shift or as you grow, and that's totally normal.

Don't worry about having a huge group. Even one or two close friends can make all the difference—quality is better than quantity. Some boys think having lots of friends is the key, but often the best moments come from hanging out with just one or two pals who really get you. As you move schools or your hobbies evolve, your squad might change. Sometimes you outgrow old friends, and that's okay, too.

Making new friends can be nerve-wracking, but there are ways to make it less stressful. Conversation starters don't have to be complicated. Try, "Hey, want to join my team?" or "Cool shirt—do you like Marvel too?" Asking what games they play or what they do after school works, too. If you're nervous, it's fine to say so: "I'm a little nervous, but I'd like to hang out." Being honest often helps people feel at ease.

Trying new lunch tables or groups can be awkward. Sometimes, people don't respond right away, but that doesn't mean you did something wrong—it just takes time. You might say, "Mind if I join you?" or "What are you guys talking about?" If it's still awkward or they're not open, don't take it personally—some groups are just set in their ways. Try another group or circle back later.

SQUAD GOALS—FRIENDSHIPS, TEASING, AND SOCIAL SUPE... | 79

Awkward moments happen to everyone—even grown-ups! If things don't work out, use humor to lighten things up or just give yourself credit for trying and move on. Every attempt makes things easier next time.

Checklist: What to Look For in a Real Friend

- Treats you with respect
- Listens and remembers what's important to you
- Shares interests or cares to learn about yours
- Makes you laugh without putting anyone down
- Has your back—even on hard days
- Celebrates your wins and supports you when things go wrong
- Doesn't pressure you to do things you're uncomfortable with
- Lets you be yourself

Friendships often start from small connections—a shared laugh, teaming up in a game, or working on a project together. Sometimes they grow online through safe chats or school platforms (with adult supervision). Other times, they begin in clubs or at practice.

If a friendship doesn't click right away, don't let it get to you. Not every try leads to a best friend. The more honest and genuine you are—sharing your real interests and listening to others—the more likely you'll find people who like being around you.

Even adults need time to find their people. Your squad will probably look different in a year, and that's all part of growing up.

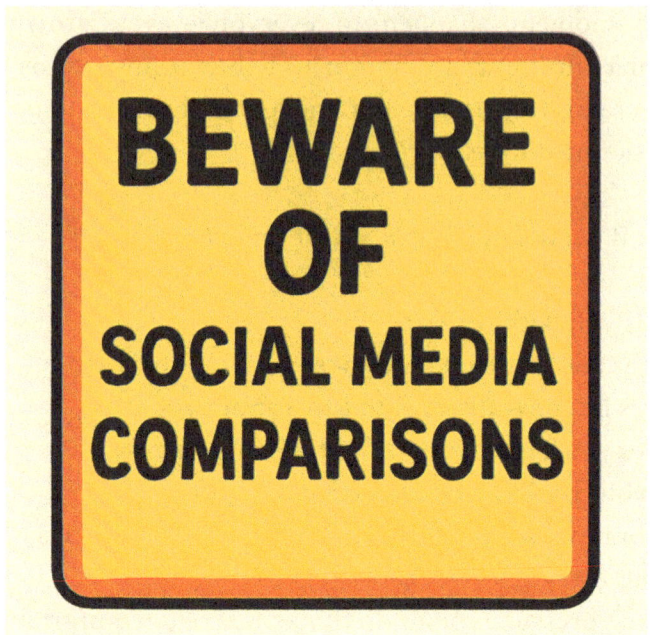

WHAT TO DO WHEN TEASING GETS REAL (SCRIPTS FOR TOUGH MOMENTS)

Teasing happens a lot in middle school and beyond. Sometimes it's harmless—a silly nickname or joke that makes everyone, including you, laugh. But sometimes, it hurts. Maybe someone comments on your voice cracking or a new pimple, and it sticks with you. It's not always clear when a joke crosses the line, but your feelings are your best guide. If you're laughing and feel good, it's probably friendly. If you feel tense, embarrassed, or left out, the teasing might have gone too far.

Spotting the difference matters. For example, if a friend jokes about your blue socks and you both laugh, that's light teasing. But if someone calls you "Smelly" every time you walk into gym and the whole class joins in, that's crossing a line. Pay attention to your gut—if you get a sinking feeling or wish you could disappear, it's a sign the teasing isn't funny anymore.

Table: Just Joking vs. Too Far—How to Tell the Difference

Just Joking	Too Far
Both laugh	Everyone laughs at you
Joke stops after you ask to stop	Joke keeps going after you ask to stop
No one feels embarrassed	Someone feels singled out, left out or embarrassed
Joke about silly stuff - (like socks)	Joke is mean - (personal or about looks)

When teasing turns mean, you don't have to deal with it alone or pretend it's okay. Strong, calm responses can work. Try saying, "That's not cool—please stop." Or, "I don't find that funny." You don't have to yell or joke back. Using a steady voice and briefly meeting their eyes shows you're serious. Sometimes, just saying, "Knock it off," is enough.

Situations can get uncomfortable fast. For instance, if someone jokes about your voice squeaking in the locker room and everyone looks at you, you have choices:

- Pause and take a breath.
- Say, "Happens to everyone."
- If they keep going, add, "Seriously, can we move on?"
- Or raise your eyebrows and ignore them—sometimes not reacting at all takes away their power.

Online group chats can also turn rough, especially if rumors start spreading. If that happens:

- Reply, "This isn't cool."
- Leave the chat for a while to let things calm down.
- Message someone you trust to talk it out. Sometimes silence is power—don't add to the drama.

If teasing keeps happening or makes you dread school, it becomes bullying. It's never embarrassing to ask for help. Telling an adult isn't tattling—it's taking care of yourself. Trusted adults like teachers, counselors, and coaches want to help. Try saying, "I need to talk about something that keeps happening," or "Someone won't leave me alone and I feel bad." They know how things like this go and want to support you.

Not sure when to get help? Here are some clues that it's time:

- Feeling nervous about school, teams, or classes.
- Being targeted repeatedly by the same person or group.
- Being left out by friends because of teasing or rumors.
- Feeling unsafe, sad, or angry most days.
- Teasing turns physical (shoving or taking things).

If any of this sounds familiar, talk to an adult you trust as soon as possible. Your feelings matter more than any joke or rumor, and often, just sharing your experience can make things start to improve.

Standing up for yourself or reaching out for support takes courage. Each time you do—whether by speaking up or just walking away—you show strength, and teach others how to treat you. If you see someone else being picked on, your support can mean a lot to them, too.

SQUAD GOALS—FRIENDSHIPS, TEASING, AND SOCIAL SUPE... | 83

Teasing can hurt, even when people say they're just joking. You deserve friends who know when to stop and who back you up when things are tough. If teasing gets to you or won't stop after you ask, use these scripts and strategies—they'll help you handle tough moments and keep your confidence strong.

PEER PRESSURE POWER-UPS—HOW TO SAY NO AND STILL BE COOL

Peer pressure is when others your age try to influence what you do —sometimes with words, other times just with looks or silence. It isn't always obvious; it might be a dare, a challenge to tease someone, or breaking a rule. Maybe it's a group sneaking out after practice, or kids sharing a video they shouldn't. It even shows up in group chats, when you feel left out for not joining in. Often, the hardest part isn't the dare itself—it's worrying you might lose your group by saying no.

I once saw my son struggle with this. At the park, his friends started teasing a quiet kid. My son wanted no part of it, but someone nudged him to join in. He knew it felt wrong but was afraid of seeming uncool. That moment happens to a lot of kids: pressure to tease, break rules, or just "fit in," even when it's wrong.

You don't have to go along to get along. Saying "no" doesn't have to be dramatic—simple phrases work: "Nah, that's not my thing," "I'm good, thanks," or "Let's do something else." These short lines are clear and don't give others much to argue with. You're not making a scene; just being honest.

Sometimes you'll need a "power-up" to shift the group. If things get mean or risky, step in with a fresh idea or a joke: "This is boring—let's play basketball instead," or, "You guys are wild. Who wants snacks?" These quick redirections help everyone move on without anyone losing face.

Humor helps a lot. If you're pressured to do something dumb, put on a silly voice and say, "I'll pass—I need my brain cells for the test," or joke, "You wish I'd do that!" Often, others are looking for an excuse to back out as well. Breaking the tension gives everyone permission to step away.

Being true to yourself is important. When you stick to what feels right, you get stronger and learn what kind of friend you want to be—one who stands up or says no, rather than just going along. That self-respect lasts longer than any joke or dare.

Sometimes, walking away is best. If people keep pushing for things that feel wrong, you don't have to stay. Say you need to leave, pretend you got a text, or just drift off. You never need a big excuse to remove yourself from a bad situation.

You can also change the direction with something positive: "Let's race to the swings," or "Who can do the best trick shot?" Suggesting a better idea gives everyone else permission to leave the negative stuff behind.

Journal Prompt: When I stood up for what I believed in...

Think of a time—big or small—where you did what felt right instead of following the crowd. Maybe you didn't laugh at a mean joke, or you spoke up for someone left out. Write about how it felt then and how you feel now.

Saying no isn't weak or boring—it's braver than nodding along. Being true to yourself is always cool. People might not notice at first, but over time, they'll remember who they can trust. You earn respect, even from those who seem annoyed at first. Holding onto your values makes you strong.

Peer pressure can be subtle. Every time you choose your path over just following the crowd, you level up. It gets easier with practice. The more you say no, change the subject, or suggest something better, the more natural it feels. If someone mocks you for not joining in, that says more about them than about you.

Being yourself is your best defense against negative pressure. Trust your gut—if something feels off, act on it. Standing alone can be tough, but those are the moments your real strength shows. The friends who stick by you when you stand up for what's right are the ones worth keeping. If someone leaves because you wouldn't join in on something wrong, they weren't really your squad.

Affirmation: Being true to myself is always cool.

DIGITAL DRAMA—HANDLING GROUP CHATS, MEMES, AND ONLINE RUMORS

Today, group chats, memes, and online jokes move fast, making it feel like you're always "on," even when you just want to relax. While digital life is mostly fun, it brings unique pressures that can creep up on you. Sometimes, a single message or meme can quickly make things awkward or hurtful.

Picture this: You're in a class group chat when someone sends an "innocent" meme. At first, it's funny—until you realize it's about a friend. The photo is embarrassing. People laugh, add emojis, and pile on with captions. The friend who's the butt of the joke might notice or might not, but you suddenly feel uneasy. Do you step in or stay quiet?

Online conversations escalate quickly. Jokes meant for a small circle can go viral in seconds. You might feel pressure to join in or stay silent so you aren't left out or labeled "uncool." But digital drama can spiral, turning jokes into real pain—it's easy to forget that what happens on screens can sting just as much as in-person teasing, and there's also a digital copy of it forever!

Before you forward, like, or post, pause and ask: Would I say this face-to-face? Would I be okay if it were about me? If you hesitate, don't send it. Remember, there's a real person on the other side—even if you're "just joking." Think about how you'd feel if your own face or mistake was meme material for everyone to see.

Checklist: "Is This Kind?"

- Would I laugh if it was about me?
- Would I show this to my grandma? Coach? Teacher?
- Would I want my name connected to this?
- Does it make anyone genuinely feel good?
- Am I proud of this now (and later)?

If there's any doubt, skip it. A quick pause can prevent a lot of drama.

When a group chat gets tense or someone tries to drag you into sharing a mean meme or rumor, there are ways to keep things cool. Try saying, "Let's not send that—it's not cool," or just steer the convo elsewhere: "Can we talk about something else?" These simple lines work better than you think. Standing up for someone online is just as important as doing it in person.

If you're targeted by mean jokes or rumors, it's tempting to clap back, but that can make things messier. Instead, take a break—mute notifications or log off for a while. If the drama continues when you're gone, take screenshots, especially if it feels like bullying.

Sometimes things get serious. If someone shares your private info, spreads rumors that won't quit, or keeps tagging you in mean posts, that's not okay. This is when it's smart to get help from an adult—not because you can't handle it, but because no one has to tackle cyberbullying alone. Parents, teachers, and counselors are there to help end it and guide you through what's next.

When to Screenshot and Talk to an Adult?

- Mean messages keep coming, even after you ask them to stop.
- A rumor gets around and people start treating you or someone else differently.
- Private pictures or info are shared without consent.
- You feel unsafe, scared, or want to avoid school or activities.
- Leaving the chat doesn't help, or people follow you to another app.

It's okay to take a break from group chats or mute them if things get overwhelming. Sometimes, stepping away for a bit can help drama settle down. There's no rule saying you have to reply instantly—come back when you're ready and things are calmer.

Screens can make drama seem huge, but you have more control than you realize. You choose what to say, who to block or mute, and when to get help from someone older. Most people want the group chat to be fun, not a source of hurt. When in doubt, pick kindness over chaos.

SUPPORTING YOUR FRIENDS—BEING AN ALLY, ON AND OFFLINE

Being an ally means looking out for others—not just sharing lunch or hanging out, but stepping in when things get uncomfortable. You might see someone always picked last or a kid left alone at recess. Noticing that is your cue to help. You don't have to be close friends with everyone, but reaching out when someone's left out is what makes you a true ally.

Standing up for others can feel awkward—your heart races and you wonder if you'll mess up or attract attention. Most kids worry about this, but doing nothing usually feels worse. If you spot someone sitting out, try a simple invitation: "Want to play?" It can feel weird, but small gestures break the ice. Even just waving someone over can make a big difference—their smile will show you that.

Being an ally also means using your voice when someone crosses a line, both in person and online. If you hear kids gossiping or making fun of someone, you can say, "Let's not talk about him like that." Or if things heat up in a group chat or game, step in with, "He's my friend, and that isn't fair." You don't need to make a scene—a calm, steady voice is enough to show kindness matters more than fitting in with mean jokes.

Supporting friends isn't just about stopping conflict. It's about checking in after tough moments, too. If your friend looks upset or leaves a game early, send a message: "You okay?" Just asking shows you care. If someone logs off suddenly, follow up later: "Saw you left—is everything alright?" It's a small gesture that reminds them they're not alone.

Friendships get stronger when you face tough stuff together.

Being an Ally Online

You'll see moments for allyship online, too. If you spot a meme targeting a classmate or mean messages being sent, don't join in or ignore it. Speak up: "Not cool—let's talk about something else." If someone's being spammed, message privately: "You don't deserve this. I'm here if you want to talk." Sometimes, not forwarding or sharing hurtful stuff is the best stand you can take.

Everyday Kindness

Kindness doesn't have to be loud. Ask someone new to join your table, your group project, or simply sit next to them and ask about their day. If reaching out feels awkward, remember everyone likes to feel included—even adults get nervous, too! Together, we can all make a better world.

When Things are Hard

If your friend faces bullies or family troubles, just being there helps. You don't have to fix everything—listening is often enough. If something feels too big for you to handle, encourage your friend to talk to a trusted adult (or help them do it). Supporting each other sometimes means sharing what's hard.

Quick Scripts for Allyship

Not sure what to say? Try:

- "Want to join us?"
- "That's my friend—please stop."
- "Are you okay?"
- "Let's do something else."

You won't get it right every time, and that's okay. Each act of allyship—big or small—builds trust and shows you're the kind of person people want on their side.

Even small kindnesses stay with people far longer than you'd think. Including someone or standing up for them doesn't just change their day—it shapes the whole environment around you for the better.

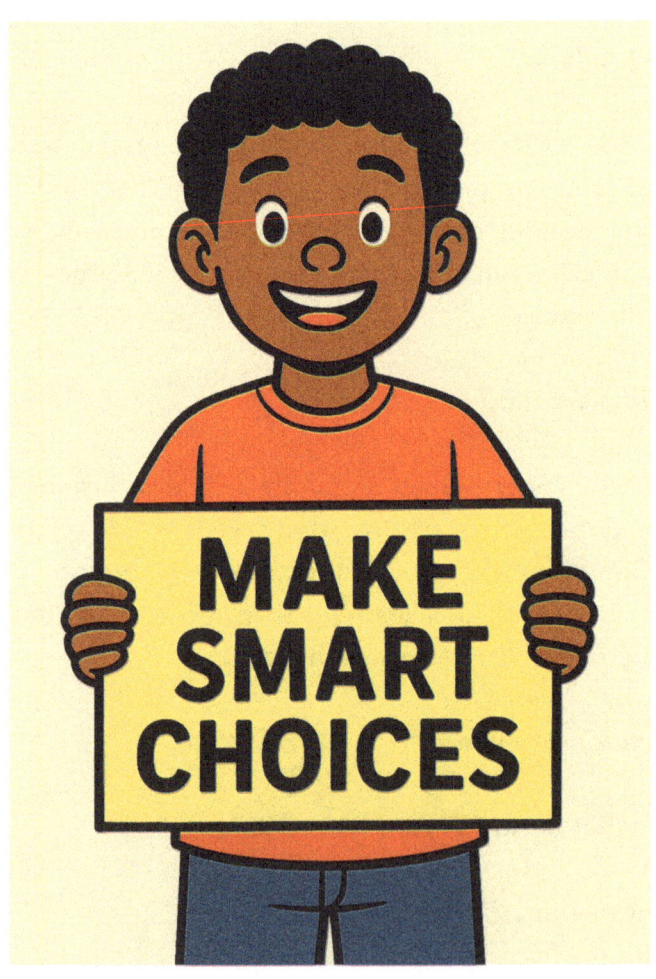

WHEN YOU FEEL LEFT OUT—REAL STRATEGIES TO BOUNCE BACK

Getting left out stings. Even if you expect it, the feeling sneaks up and makes your stomach twist. Maybe you saw photos from a party you weren't invited to, or watched a group walk away while you pretended not to care. That invisible feeling is normal—everyone, even the most confident, has been there. I once talked with a boy who missed a sleepover and spent the weekend upset, convinced nobody liked him. Later, he found out another friend wasn't invited either. They hung out together and had a surprisingly good time, once they gave themselves the chance.

Reactions to being left out can be dramatic. Some get angry and snap at the group; others withdraw and shut everyone out. The urge to make a dramatic exit or post online can be strong, but it rarely helps. Lashing out usually makes things worse. Staying isolated can turn a small hurt into a big one, and you may miss out on new opportunities. Instead, give yourself space to feel bad—cry, punch a pillow, or just admit it stinks—but then, try to bounce back.

A helpful trick is to make a list of things you enjoy solo: building models, drawing, shooting hoops, coding, or just watching funny videos. Solo time can be fun and sometimes leads you to others who share your interests—through clubs, online (safely), or just around the neighborhood.

After cooling off, try reaching out to someone new instead of waiting for an invite. Maybe there's a classmate outside your main group you can ask: "Want to hang out after school?" or "Can I join your game?" It takes guts, but most people are open, they may just be waiting for someone to reach out first.

Talking about feeling left out is important. Bottling it up doesn't help. Start small: "I felt kind of left out today. Can we talk?" This works with friends, parents, teachers, or anyone you trust. Most adults remember the feeling and will listen. Sometimes just saying it out loud eases the burden.

If you feel ready, you can ask your group directly: "Hey, I noticed I wasn't invited last time. Did I do something?" Usually, it isn't personal; maybe there was limited space, or they forgot. But if you're repeatedly excluded on purpose, that's a sign they may not be real friends.

Self-compassion is key. Don't blame yourself or assume the worst. Try to reframe: instead of "Nobody wants me," think, "Today was tough, but it's just one day." Find something positive; time to do what you enjoy, or to get closer to someone new.

Bounce-Back Checklist

1. Let yourself feel sad or annoyed—then do something you enjoy.
2. Reach out to someone new or spend time with family.
3. Talk about it with someone who listens.

Affirmation Reminder

"One left-out day doesn't define me." It's just one event, not your whole story.

Social situations are always shifting. Groups change, friendships move around, and the kid who feels left out today might be including others tomorrow. Everyone misses out sometimes—even adults. Your feelings are valid.

Keep busy. Dive into hobbies, help someone else who may feel left out, or try something new. Helping others can also lift your own mood.

With time, resilience grows. Each time you bounce back, you get stronger. You start seeing that missing one event isn't the end—and often opens up new possibilities.

If you feel invisible or unwanted, know you're not alone. Everyone experiences this—even those who seem to have it all together. What matters is how you respond: try new things, talk about your feelings, and reach out to others.

Friendships are always evolving, and no one gets through middle school without bumps. Each hard moment proves you're learning more about yourself and others. Next up? Taking care of your body and mind so you can keep showing up for yourself—and your friends—no matter what comes next.

6

FUEL, REST, AND STRENGTH—TAKING CARE OF YOUR CHANGING BODY

EAT LIKE A CHAMP—WHAT TO SNACK ON (AND WHAT TO SKIP)

Think of your body as a race car; you wouldn't fill a race car with soda and expect it to win. The fuel you choose is what keeps you energized, helps you grow, and keeps your brain sharp, whether you're in a big game or taking a test. During puberty, your body is working harder than ever—building new muscles, bones, and even brain cells. Eating well has never been more important.

What you eat can make a big difference in how you feel and perform. Candy bars may give a quick sugar rush, but that energy fades fast and might leave you feeling tired or cranky. Balanced meals and snacks keep your energy steady, helping you focus in class, power through practice, or just get through the day without crashing. Think of eating as charging your phone—good food means a fully charged battery for whatever comes next.

A balanced plate—or "Power Plate"—is simple: Fill half with fruits and veggies (the more colorful, the better), and the other half with protein (chicken, eggs, tofu, or beans) and carbs (rice, pasta, or bread). Add a small portion of healthy fat from nuts or cheese, for meat-free eaters, beans or tofu work great. Mixing things up keeps meals interesting and makes sure your body gets all the tools it needs to grow.

Snacking is normal, especially if you're busy, but not all snacks are equal. Go for snacks that keep you full and energized, not ones that lead to a crash. Examples: apples with peanut butter, string cheese with whole-grain crackers, or yogurt with berries. These choices provide protein and lasting energy—unlike candy or soda, which can spike and drop your blood sugar. If you want crunch, try air-popped popcorn instead of chips. For a sweet fix, grab fruit rather than candy.

Don't skip breakfast—it really does help you get through the morning. Something simple like oatmeal, a banana with nut butter, or trail mix can jumpstart your day and help you focus until lunch. If mornings are rushed, set out snacks the night before so they're easy to grab on the go.

Eating out with friends means lots of tempting choices, but you don't have to give up favorites. Balance is what matters. If everyone's ordering burgers, add a side salad or swap fries for apple slices. At pizza places, choose veggie toppings or thin crust if possible. With fast food, grilled is usually better than fried, and water is better than soda.

It's normal to be picky about food at your age. Tastes change, so foods you dislike now might become favorites later. If you're stuck eating the same things, simple changes—like grilling instead of boiling—can make a big difference in flavor.

SNACK SWAP: SMART CHOICES FOR BUSY DAYS

Snack Swap	
Potato Chips	Popcorn - Air Popped
Candy	Apple or Banana
Soda	Water or Milk
Fried Chicken Nuggets	Grilled Chicken Strips
Sugary Cereal	Oatmeal with Fruit
Packaged Pastries	Yogurt with Berries

For busy days, pack grab-and-go snacks like trail mix, low-sugar granola bars, pre-sliced fruit, cheese sticks, nuts (if allowed), hard-boiled eggs, or veggie sticks to help you feel full and fueled.

Food is fuel, not just something to eat when bored or stressed. Eating well helps you build strong bones and muscles, and keeps your brain sharp.. Treats are fine sometimes—birthday cake has its place! But if most of your snacks are from bright packages or fast food, try swapping some for "power foods."

If you need new snack ideas or want help with school lunches, talk to someone at home. You might discover new foods you enjoy and get others to join you in trying something different! Maybe it's time for you to explore the kitchen and try cooking as your new hobby or passion.

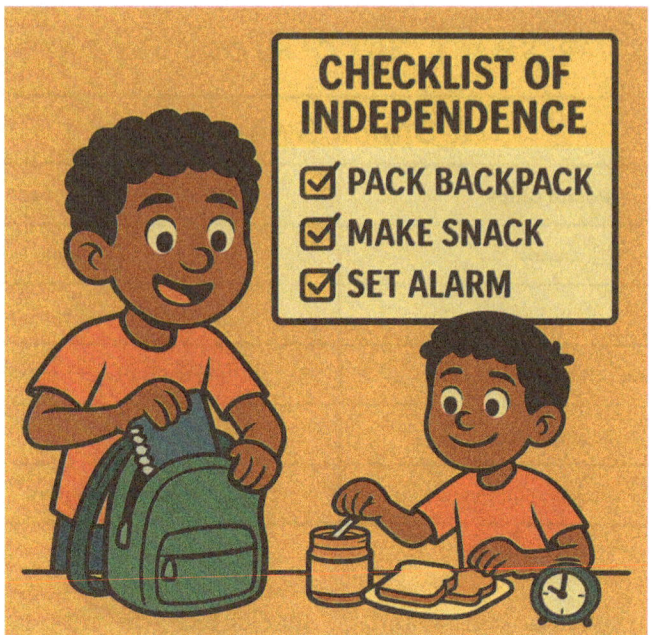

THIRST TRAP—WHY WATER IS YOUR SECRET SUPERPOWER

You probably don't think much about water as you rush through the day. Maybe you grab a juice box or a sports drink, or you just forget about drinks until you're super thirsty and your mouth feels like the desert. But here's the thing: your body needs water all the time, not just after running around or on a hot day. Water is like your body's secret fuel. It helps every part of you work better—your muscles, your brain, even your mood. Think of yourself like a plant. Plants wilt and droop if you skip watering them, no matter how sunny the window. Your body works the same way. You need steady sips to stand tall, stay sharp, and keep growing strong.

When you're in a growth spurt, your body works overtime to stretch bones, build muscle, and keep your skin healthy. That means you use up more water than usual. Add sports or hot days, and it's even easier to run dry. Most of the time, you don't notice you're getting dehydrated until your body shouts at you—headaches out of nowhere, feeling tired when you shouldn't, trouble focusing in class, or just feeling grumpy for no reason. Sometimes you get dizzy or notice your pee is really dark yellow instead of pale. When that happens, your body is waving a red flag saying, "Hey! I'm thirsty!" If you ignore it, it just gets worse—more tiredness, crankiness, and sometimes even stomachaches or muscle cramps.

So, how do you know if you're getting enough water? It's not rocket science. If you're thirsty, you're already on the low side. If your mouth is dry or your lips feel cracked, your body is sending warning signals. Feeling tired during the day for no good reason? Another sign. If you get headaches after gym or find yourself struggling to pay attention at school, water might be the fix. Even feeling oddly hungry can sometimes mean you're actually thirsty.

Checklist: Are You Drinking Enough?

- Does your mouth feel dry after recess or gym?
- Are you getting headaches during the day?
- Do you feel tired even when you slept well?
- Is your pee dark yellow instead of light?
- Do you forget to drink during class or after sports?

If you said yes to more than one, it might be time to up your water game.

Staying hydrated isn't hard once it becomes a habit. Start simple. Carry a water bottle everywhere—school, practice, even in the car. Choose one with cool designs or stickers that make you want to use it. Set a goal to finish and refill it at least three times a day. Some bottles have lines showing how much to drink by different times (like "Drink to this line by lunch!"). If yours doesn't, draw your own with a marker or tape. Phones and smartwatches can help, too—set short reminders for a quick sip every hour or so.

Not everyone loves plain water, and that's okay. You can jazz it up without loading up on sugar. Drop in slices of lemon or lime, toss in frozen berries for a burst of color and taste, or add a splash of 100% fruit juice for fun flavor. Some kids like cucumber slices or even a sprig of mint for something different. If it looks cool and tastes good, you're more likely to drink up.

There are sneaky ways to get more water, too—eat foods that contain a lot of water! Crunchy snacks like watermelon, oranges, cucumbers, strawberries, and celery are tasty and count toward hydration. Pair them with lunch or as an after-school snack to help out your body without even thinking about it.

Water beats soda or energy drinks every time—those only make you thirstier later and fill you with sugar that leads to an energy crash. Milk is good for meals, but nothing beats plain water for everyday hydration. Don't wait until you feel thirsty; sip during class changes, after every bathroom break, and before and after sports.

It's easy to forget about water when life gets busy, but sticking with it pays off big time. You'll notice better focus, steadier moods, smoother skin, and fewer headaches. And if you ever find yourself dragging through the day for no reason, try drinking a tall glass of water—sometimes it's all you need to bounce back fast.

Drinking enough isn't just for athletes or kids who play outside all day. Even if your favorite activity is gaming or reading comics on the couch, your brain needs water to keep up with all that thinking and learning. So next time someone asks what your superpower is, tell them: "Staying hydrated!" Because honestly, it makes everything else possible.

MOVE YOUR BODY—SPORTS, EXERCISE, AND JUST HAVING FUN

Most people talk about sports as if they're only for future pros or the "athletic" kids. Here's the truth: moving your body isn't just for athletes. It's for everyone, even if you're more into comics or building epic LEGO sets than joining a team. Being active helps you in more ways than you might expect. Regular movement boosts your mood, builds confidence, and helps your body grow stronger and healthier. You don't have to win medals or play on a team to get these benefits. Just moving every day—however you want—makes a huge difference.

Maybe you love the idea of basketball with friends, or perhaps you'd rather skateboard alone at the park. There's no right way to get moving. Some kids love hiking or running with their dog. Others dance in their rooms when nobody's watching. You might enjoy biking around your neighborhood, bouncing on a trampoline, climbing trees, or chasing your little brother at the playground. Even things like walking to school, shoveling snow, or mowing the lawn count as real exercise. On rainy days, challenge yourself with YouTube fitness routines or try out silly dance videos. If you have a friend or sibling who will play dodgeball or kickball with you, that works too. You can even make up new games—think "how many jumping jacks can I do before my favorite song ends?" or "can I beat my best time running around the block?"

Don't buy into the idea that you have to be "good" at something to enjoy it. Everyone starts somewhere, and nobody looks cool the first time they try something new. Remember that kid who wiped out on his skateboard but kept laughing and got right back up? Or the one who tried Zumba with his aunt and looked like a confused octopus? They had fun anyway and actually got better just by showing up and moving. You don't need a uniform or fancy gear. Just pick something that sounds fun and give it a go.

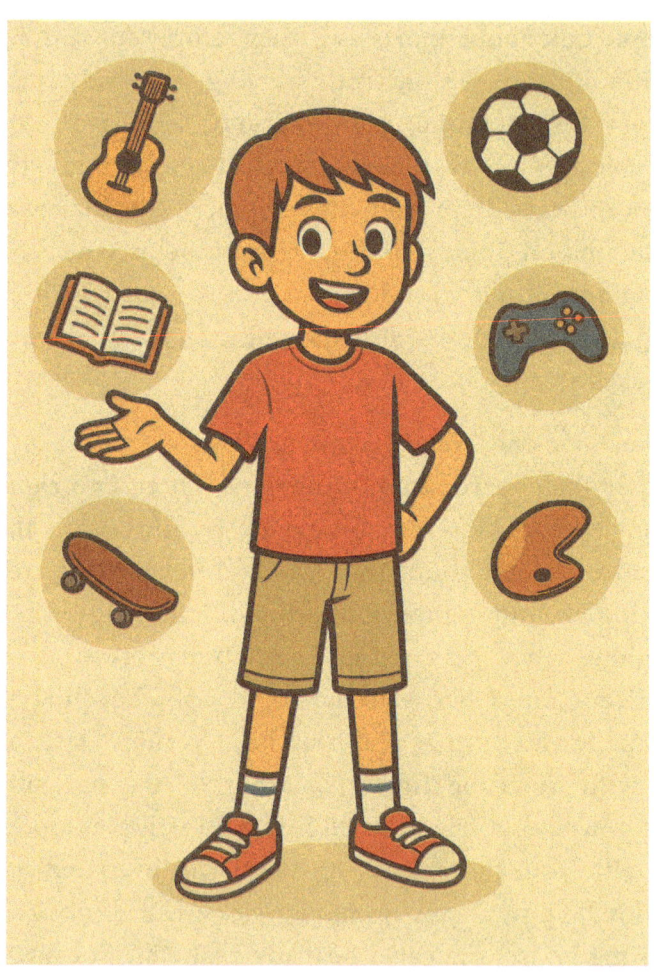

Moving your body does more than just make you stronger. It can make a rough day feel lighter. Exercise kicks stress to the curb by letting your brain release "feel-good" chemicals—kind of like natural happy juice for your mind. Sometimes, after a tough day at school or a fight with a friend, going for a walk or shooting hoops can help melt away some of the anger or sadness. I remember when my grandson felt down after a bad day; he started taking daily bike rides around our block. He didn't train for anything special, just pedaled until his thoughts got quieter and he could breathe easier again.

Movement also helps you sleep better at night. Even if you just go outside for 10 minutes to stretch or toss a ball around, your body gets tired in a good way. This makes it easier to fall asleep and wake up ready for a new day. And believe it or not, staying active can even help your skin. When you sweat, your body gets rid of stuff it doesn't need, which can help keep pimples away (as long as you wash up after).

Don't let embarrassment stop you from trying new things. Nobody is born knowing how to do every move or play every sport. The best way to discover what you like is by trying things out, even if you feel awkward at first. You might surprise yourself and end up loving something you never expected—like martial arts, yoga, or shooting baskets in your driveway after dinner.

Not everyone likes big crowds or noisy teams, and that's totally fine. If you'd rather move solo, there are tons of ways to stay active on your own. Try jump rope challenges, skateboarding tricks, or see how many times you can bounce a ball in a row without dropping it. If you're more social, invite friends for weekend pickup games, bike rides, or even walks around the mall.

If sticking with one thing gets boring fast, switch it up! Make your own "try-it" challenge: pick a new activity each month and see what sticks. One month could involve swimming at the local pool, while the next month might be spent hiking with family or learning a TikTok dance routine. Keep track of what makes you smile or helps you shake off stress.

The most important thing is to move every day in some way that feels good to you, not what someone else says you "should" do. Whether you're goofy, quiet, competitive, or just curious, your body will thank you for every step, jump, pedal, and dance move.

SLEEP HACKS—GETTING ENOUGH REST IN A BUSY WORLD

Puberty throws your sleep out of whack—one minute you're dozing off early, the next you're wide awake at midnight and can barely get up for school. Your body is working hard, growing bones and muscles, and wiring your brain for tougher challenges and bigger feelings. Sleep is your body's repair shop: it recharges you, fixes what needs fixing, and sweeps out the mental clutter of the day. Without enough rest, you get cranky, think less clearly, and even little challenges feel overwhelming. School gets harder, your mood shifts quickly, and you can get sick more easily.

But in real life, good sleep doesn't just happen. Schedules are busy—after-school stuff, homework, group chats pinging late, and FOMO (Fear Of Missing Out) if you log off first. Screens make it harder to snooze. The bright light from phones and tablets tricks your brain into thinking it's daytime, and gaming or videos can keep your mind buzzing. Late sports or family plans push bedtime back, too. And once you finally lie down, worries can pop up—about school, awkward moments, or just random things your brain invents. All these steal your sleep.

You can outsmart these with some simple tricks. Set a "screen curfew"—turn off gadgets at least 30 minutes before bed (your brain will thank you). Need your phone as an alarm? Put it across the room so you won't scroll. Dim your room's lights to help your body ease into "sleep mode." If your mind races, keep a notebook by your bed and write down your thoughts or worries. Sometimes, just jotting them down lets your brain rest.

A bedtime routine signals to your body it's time to slow down. Keep it simple and follow it nightly, even on weekends. Brush your teeth, wash up, then pick something relaxing (not screens!). Read, doodle, or draw; listen to chill music or a podcast with dim lights; stretch your muscles. If you share your room or it's noisy, try earplugs or ask for ten minutes of quiet before bed.

5 Steps to a Chill Bedtime

1. Turn off all screens 30 minutes before bed.
2. Brush teeth, wash face, and put on pajamas.
3. Dim the lights and tidy up any mess.
4. Read, draw, stretch, or listen to calm music.
5. Climb into bed at the same time every night—even weekends.

Even with good habits, you may still toss and turn or wake up at 3 AM. That's normal now and then. If you have a bad night, don't panic or force yourself to sleep—that backfires. Try something quiet, such as reading or gentle music, with the lights dimmed. Avoid checking the clock; it only makes it harder.

If you're tired the next morning, do what helps you get by until bed—have some breakfast, move around outside if you can, and let people know if you're having a tough day. Avoid loading up on sugar or energy drinks. They'll give a short boost but make the crash worse.

Nobody sleeps perfectly every night—not even adults. The key is to shake off bad nights and not let them become habits. Stick to your routine and give yourself credit for trying new ways to relax.

If worries or sleeplessness become frequent, talk to someone at home or school. Sharing what's on your mind can help.

Puberty alters the amount and timing of sleep needed. Trust your body—it knows what it's doing. Give yourself the rest you need so you're ready for what comes next: new classes, bigger feelings, taller mornings, and maybe even better dreams (even the weird ones about flying llamas or zombie teachers).

IS LIFTING WEIGHTS SAFE? BUSTING FITNESS MYTHS FOR PRETEENS

You might hear, "Don't lift weights or you'll stop growing!" or "Working out is only for older kids." These myths simply aren't true if you're careful. Old ideas that lifting weights hurts kids' growth plates have been disproven—science shows that with safe moves, good form, and adult guidance, strength training is not only safe for preteens but actually beneficial. It strengthens muscles, bones, and even helps your brain as you grow.

But don't try to lift like a superhero. No one wants you bench pressing cars or mimicking pro wrestlers. Safe strength training for preteens means using bodyweight or light resistance that you can control easily. If you strain too much or feel like you're forcing a move, it's too heavy. Focus on exercises that make you stronger for daily activities, not just for looks.

Start with bodyweight exercises—these use your weight as resistance, so you don't need dumbbells or machines. Push-ups (or wall push-ups if regular ones are too hard) work your arms and chest. Squats target your legs and glutes. Planks build core strength, and wall sits work your thighs and are fun to do with friends. Resistance bands are another safe addition; they challenge your muscles while being gentle on your joints, provided you use them with slow, controlled movements.

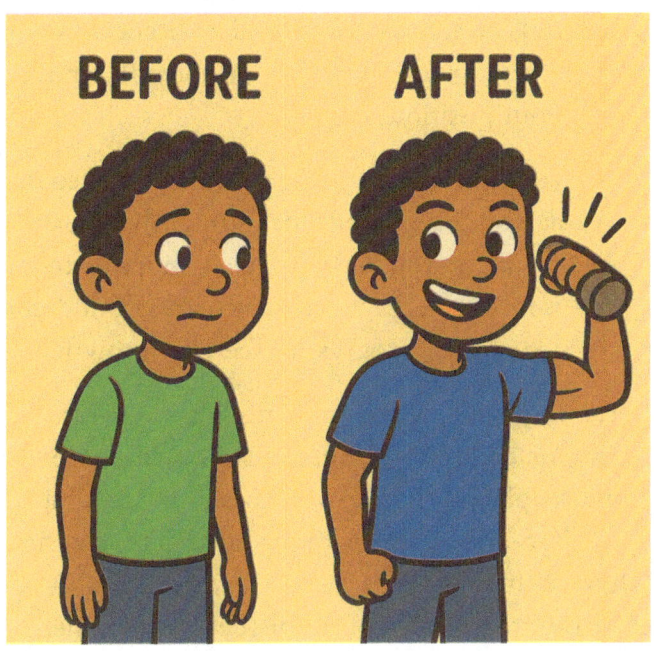

No gym membership or special equipment is required—just some space and possibly a wall. Always warm up before you start. Ten jumping jacks, big arm circles, and gentle stretching get your blood flowing and prepare your muscles. Think of warming up like prepping your game console—it's important so everything runs smoothly.

When trying new moves, ask an adult to check your form. Parents, siblings, coaches, or gym teachers can see if you're at risk of injury. Good form matters more than the number of reps or how much weight you lift. If you experience sharp pain, especially in your joints, stop immediately and seek advice from a knowledgeable person.

Here's a starter list of safe moves: regular or wall push-ups, squats (feet shoulder-width apart, sit back as if into a chair), planks (body straight on elbows and toes), wall sits (back flat to the wall, knees bent as if sitting), and resistance band stretches. You can find videos for these, but always listen to your body. If a move feels off, stop and check your position.

Set small, realistic goals and build up gradually. You could start by holding a plank for 20 seconds or doing five push-ups. The following week, add a rep or try for a more extended hold. Celebrate tiny improvements each week—these build confidence fast. Keep a record of your progress to see your growth over time.

Strength training isn't about out-muscling others. It's about building skills for daily life—climbing stairs with ease, carrying a heavy backpack, playing harder at recess, or standing taller for class photos. For added motivation, consider starting a "mini workout club" with a friend or family member. You can challenge each other or race to hold a wall sit for the longest time.

Above all, pay attention to your body. If you're tired, it's okay to rest—recovery is part of getting stronger. Don't force extra reps if you feel shaky or sore in a bad way. Learn to tell the difference between normal tiredness and pain. When in doubt, ask an adult before trying something new.

You won't see big muscles overnight, and that's normal. Physical changes come with time, especially as you hit puberty, but real strength comes through sticking with your routine and enjoying the process. Notice small improvements, like easier squats or longer plank holds; these are true signs of progress, even if others can't see them yet.

To mix things up, join beginner fitness classes at your community center or school—try yoga, martial arts, dance, or strength classes designed for kids. These are fun and safe ways to learn new moves and receive feedback on your form.

The most important thing is to keep strength activities fun and focused on feeling good, not getting "huge" or comparing yourself to others. Choose moves that challenge you without hurting, look for steady improvement, and always prioritize safety. Building strength now helps not just in sports or classes, but also for chores and all the moments when you need a little extra muscle power in daily life.

ENERGY SLUMPS—HOW TO RECHARGE WITHOUT SUGAR BOMBS

Energy crashes sneak up on you. One minute, you're feeling fine, maybe even bouncing off the walls. The next, you're slumped at your desk, staring at the clock and wondering how you'll make it to the end of class. This is not just a "you" thing—it happens to everyone, especially during puberty. There are a bunch of reasons you might feel wiped out, and most don't have anything to do with being lazy. Skipping meals, forgetting to drink water, sitting for hours on end, or staring at screens for too long can all make your energy tank. Sometimes, it's all of these together that hit you hardest right after lunch or when the afternoon drags on forever.

I remember a boy named Ryan who always felt tired after lunch. He'd eat a huge plate of fries and wash it down with a soda because he thought the sugar would keep him awake for math class. Instead, he'd end up with his head on his desk, struggling to listen. At first, he thought he just wasn't a "school person," but after a few changes—like eating an apple with peanut butter instead of candy and drinking water instead of soda—he started feeling less sleepy. He also started taking stretch breaks and noticed he didn't zone out as much in class. Small changes made his afternoons better.

So what actually works when you hit that wall? If you catch yourself yawning or losing focus, try standing up and stretching your arms above your head or rolling your shoulders. Move your legs and take a quick walk, even if it's just to refill your water bottle. Step outside for two minutes of fresh air if you can. These tiny moves wake up your body and brain faster than you'd think. If you can't leave your seat, even wiggling your toes or flexing your fingers helps. Your body needs movement as much as it needs food and water for energy.

Drinking water is another game-changer. It's easy to forget, but even slight dehydration can cause your mind to feel foggy and your muscles to feel heavy. When school or homework gets tough, take a few big sips before reaching for anything else. If you're hungry, grab a snack that has protein and some carbs, like a piece of cheese with crackers or yogurt with fruit. These keep your energy up longer than candy or chips.

Now, remember about those sugar bombs—candy bars, soda, energy drinks—they promise quick power, but it's all smoke and mirrors. Sugar gives you a fast jolt of energy because it surges into your blood super quickly. You feel hyped for about 30 minutes, maybe less. Then comes the crash: your energy drops even lower than before, leaving you tired, cranky, and sometimes even hungrier than when you started. This up-and-down cycle can make you feel like a yo-yo all day long. Energy drinks are even worse because they also have caffeine, which makes falling asleep harder later. If you reach for these all the time, it's easy to get stuck in a loop of short bursts followed by long slumps.

A better plan is to set yourself up with small habits that help you avoid feeling drained in the first place. Schedule breaks during homework or study time to stand up and move every 20–30 minutes. Keep snacks like trail mix or an apple in your backpack so you're not tempted by vending machines when hunger hits. Make it a habit to have water nearby and sip it throughout the day, instead of chugging all at once after gym or at dinner.

You can also do "energy check-ins" at different times of day. Ask yourself: Did I eat breakfast? Have I moved around in the last hour? How much water have I had? Noticing patterns can help you see what makes you feel good and what leaves you dragging. If you realize screens zap your energy after a while, set a timer for breaks or switch to something active before returning to your game.

Long-lasting energy comes from taking care of your whole self: moving around, eating snacks that last, drinking enough water, and knowing when to hit pause on screens or homework for just five minutes of movement or stretching. It's not about being perfect—everyone will have days when they feel wiped out—but building these habits gives you more control over how you feel.

When you know how to recharge without reaching for sugar bombs or another soda, you'll notice days go smoother and your mood stays steadier. You'll be awake enough to enjoy the fun stuff and focused enough to get through the boring parts, too. Even little tweaks—like adding an extra stretch break or swapping one snack—can change how you feel by the end of the day.

No chapter on caring for your body is complete without discussing recharging, right? From smart snacks to quick movement breaks and skipping those fake sugar boosts, these moves help keep your body running strong during all the wild changes of puberty. Remember, what you think and feel shapes who you become as much as any snack or workout ever could.

Next up: we'll talk about, Real Talk Q & A—honest answers to your toughest questions.

7

REAL TALK Q&A—HONEST ANSWERS TO YOUR TOUGHEST QUESTIONS

ERECTIONS EXPLAINED—WHY THEY HAPPEN (AND WHAT TO DO)

Picture this: you're in the middle of math, bored out of your mind, and all of a sudden, your body decides to make things interesting—boom—an erection. You didn't think about anything weird or exciting. You didn't even move. Yet there it is, and you're just hoping nobody notices while the teacher asks you to come up to the board. This is one of those classic puberty moments that almost every boy worries about but nobody talks about out loud. If you've ever wondered what's up with these surprise body reactions, you're definitely not alone.

So, what is an erection? It's when the penis gets hard and a little bigger because blood rushes in and fills it up. It's not like there's a bone inside (that's a myth—no bones here, just blood flow). This is a totally normal part of puberty and growing up. Your body is loaded with new hormones right now—think of them as messages zooming around telling different parts to grow, change, or act in new ways. Sometimes, these messages get sent even if you're not doing anything special or thinking about anything in particular. It's kind of like getting goose bumps or having hiccups. Erections can happen automatically, just because your body feels like it.

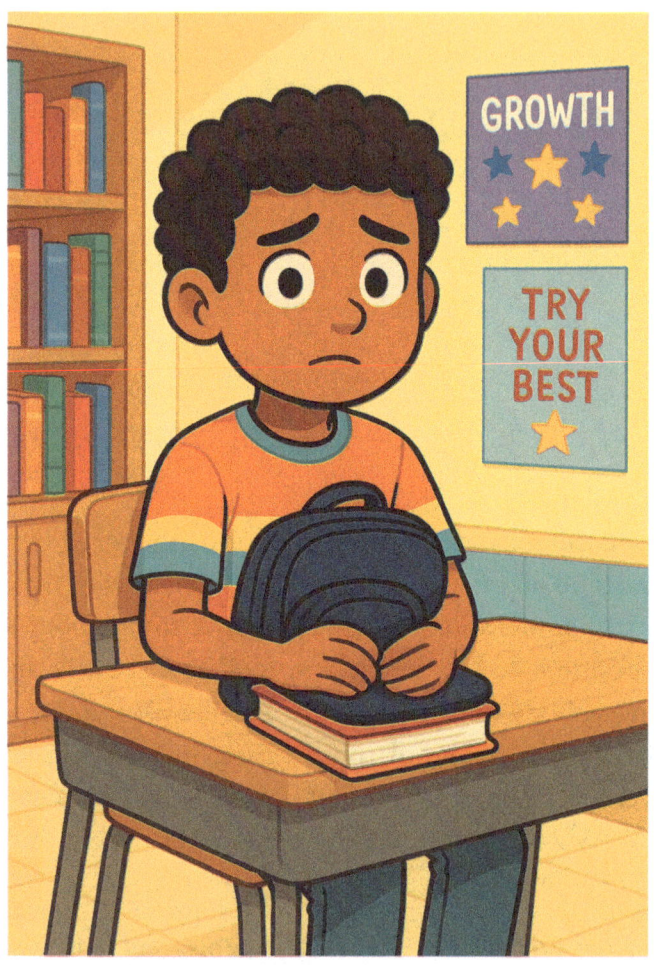

Here's the wild part—not every erection is about what you're thinking. Sure, sometimes it might happen if you have a crush or see something that makes your heart race. However, they also appear at the most unexpected times. You could be watching cartoons, walking the dog, riding the bus, or just waking up in the morning. There's no "right" or "wrong" time for your body to do this. It doesn't mean anything is wrong with you if it happens a lot, or even if it happens when you don't want it to. Your body is just practicing for future grown-up stuff. You can't always control when an erection starts or stops, which is why they sometimes show up at the most annoying times.

Feeling embarrassed? You're not the only one. Many boys worry that someone will notice or say something. The truth is, most people are way too busy with their own lives to see what's going on under your desk or behind your backpack. Clothes usually hide everything anyway. Most erections only last a few minutes and then fade away. Here are some tricks that guys use—sit down and wait it out, put a book or backpack on your lap, wear longer shirts if you're nervous about school days. If you get called to stand up and it won't go away right away, try tucking the waistband of your underwear over the top to keep things hidden (it sounds silly, but it works for some). Focus on something boring or count backward from one hundred to take your mind off things.

Let's bust a few myths while we're at it. Some people say, "If you get too many erections, something is wrong with you." That's just not true. During puberty, it's normal for boys to have lots of them —even several in a day—because hormones are basically learning how to do their job. Another rumor is that "everyone will notice." Nope! Unless you're wearing superhero tights with no pants over them, your jeans or shorts are doing their job. Plus, almost nobody pays as much attention as you think they do.

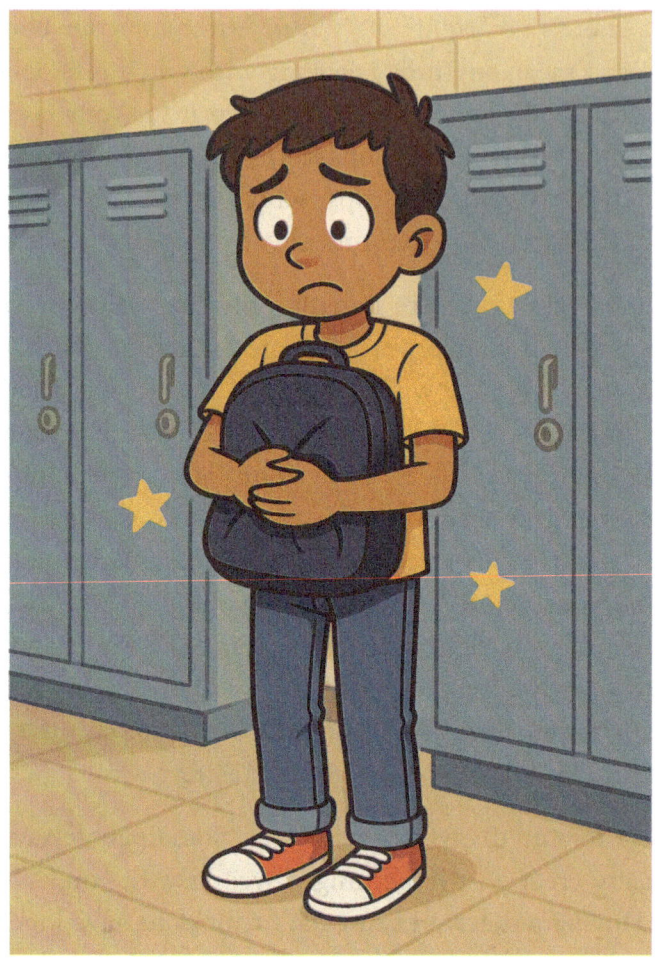

Ready for a little Q&A?

- **Q: Do erections mean I'm weird or doing something wrong?**
    - A: Not at all. They are automatic—sometimes they show up for no reason at all.
- **Q: Can I stop myself from getting an erection?**
    - A: Not really. You can sometimes distract yourself or think about something else if you feel one coming on, but your body still runs the show.

- **Q: Is it bad if I get an erection a lot?**
  - A: No! It's just your body practicing.
- **Q: Can other people tell?**
  - A: Almost never. Regular clothes keep everything private.

Try This: "Erection Panic Survival Kit"

Make a mental checklist for those surprise moments:

1. Sit down and wait—most go away in a minute or two.
2. Use your backpack, jacket, or folder as a shield.
3. Wear longer shirts on days when you feel extra nervous.
4. Breathe slow and focus on something else.
5. Remind yourself—every guy goes through this.

Remember, you're not alone. These things can feel awkward but are just proof your body is working like it should. If you have questions that feel too weird to ask anyone in your family, write them down or talk to an adult you trust later on. There's nothing shameful or strange about your body doing its thing—even if it picks the most random times possible!

WET DREAMS 101—WHAT'S NORMAL AND WHY IT'S NOT WEIRD

Waking up to find your pajamas or sheets damp and sticky can be surprising or worrying, but if this happens to you, you've experienced what's called a wet dream. Wet dreams are completely normal and common during puberty. They occur when your body releases semen while you're asleep—sometimes during a dream, and sometimes with no dream at all. Just like getting new body hair or your voice changing, wet dreams are simply another sign that your body is growing up and hormones are doing their thing.

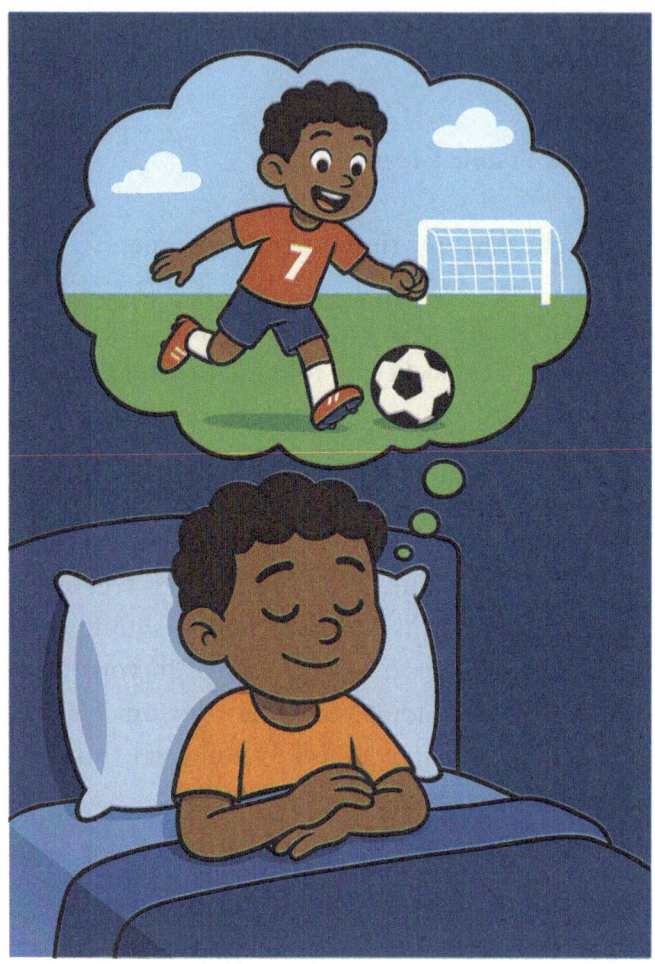

You don't choose to have wet dreams, and you can't control or prevent them. Some boys have them a lot, some just a few times, and some might not notice them at all—there's no "normal" amount. Wet dreams don't say anything about your thoughts, personality, or whether you're weird or abnormal. It's just your body adjusting to puberty, and there's nothing to be ashamed of or feel guilty about—think of it like sneezing in your sleep: unplanned, but normal.

If you realize you've had a wet dream, remember: you did nothing wrong. There's no reason to feel guilty, dirty, or embarrassed. Most boys will have at least one wet dream during puberty, and it happens worldwide to boys your age, even if nobody talks about it.

What should you do after a wet dream? Simply change into some clean pajamas or underwear. If your sheets are messy, pull them off the bed and put them in the laundry. To keep things private, you can wait until no one's around, wrap up the sheets, or do your own laundry if possible. If you need to ask for help, you could just say, "My bed got messy last night—can we wash my sheets?" Trust that most adults have dealt with much stranger situations!

It's normal if you need to wash your pajamas too. If privacy is a concern, consider doing your laundry by yourself or ask someone to show you how to use the washer. Every family is different—some talk about this openly, others don't—but remember, wet dreams are just part of growing up.

Let's clear up a few common myths: First, it's false that only certain boys get wet dreams—boys everywhere, from all backgrounds, may have them at different times during puberty. Second, you can't stop or control wet dreams no matter how hard you try. They're automatic and happen without your choice, so having more (or fewer) than others doesn't mean anything is wrong.

If you're worried whether you're having wet dreams too often or not at all, know that everyone's experience is different—some might have a few a month, others go months without any. Wet dreams usually become less frequent as you get older, but sometimes continue into adulthood, and none of this means anything about your health or who you are.

If you ever feel uneasy talking about wet dreams at home, that's okay. Write your questions down or talk to someone you trust—a parent, sibling, coach, counselor, or doctor. Remember, most adults know about wet dreams, even if it's not something that's often discussed. If you ever have unusual symptoms—like pain, blood, or odd smells—see a doctor just to be safe.

Bottom line: wet dreams are nothing to be ashamed of. They don't define you, aren't a sign of something wrong, and no one can tell if you've had one. Like sudden growth or a changing voice, wet dreams are part of puberty. Take care of cleanup in a way that feels comfortable, and know that this is totally normal and nothing to worry about.

WHAT'S THE DEAL WITH MASTURBATION?

Okay, let's talk about something that might feel a little weird to bring up, but it's totally normal to wonder about. During puberty, your body starts responding to all kinds of new feelings and sensations. Sometimes you might notice that touching your private parts feels good. That's called masturbation—and yep, it's something many guys try as they grow up.

Some boys do it, some don't. It's a personal choice. You're not "weird" if you're curious, and you're not "behind" if you're not. It's private—not something to talk about in the locker room or show off about. It's just one of those body things that some people explore in their own time, in their own space.

Masturbation doesn't mean something's wrong with you. It's not dangerous, it won't hurt you, and it's not something you need to feel guilty about. It's your body figuring stuff out—kind of like testing the controls on a new machine. The important thing? It should always be private and respectful—something you only do when you're alone, in a safe space.

Still not sure how to feel about it? That's okay. If you have questions, write them down or talk to someone you trust when you're ready. Puberty brings a lot of new experiences—this is just one of them. No shame, no panic. Just real talk.

"WHY AM I GROWING AT MY OWN PACE?"—THE SCIENCE OF BEING DIFFERENT

Ever look at a group photo and wonder why you seem so different from your friends or cousins? Maybe someone's already taller than his dad or growing a mustache in sixth grade, while you feel like your body missed a memo. Here's the truth—growing up happens at different speeds for everyone, and there's solid science behind it.

A lot of it comes down to your family tree. Genetics act as a secret code, influencing your height, when your voice deepens, and when you start getting new hair. If you flip through old pictures of your dad, uncles, or grandpa at your age, you might notice a pattern—some families have late bloomers, some early. It's not just what you eat or how much you sleep. Hormones do most of the work. These chemical messengers get busy during puberty, triggering all sorts of changes: new muscles, taller height, a deeper voice, new hair, even mood swings. The catch is, timing is different for everyone—even twin brothers can develop at totally different rates.

So, it's normal to feel out of sync with your friends. Some boys get called "shrimp" or "beanpole," while others are ducking under door frames when no one else has even started growing yet. It's common to feel like you're last in line. One boy I remember was always the smallest in his group—picked last for teams, tired of the jokes, always struggling on the basketball court. Then, at the end of eighth grade, he suddenly shot up and by high school was the tallest on his team. The teasing stopped fast. Changes can sneak up on you, sometimes when you least expect it.

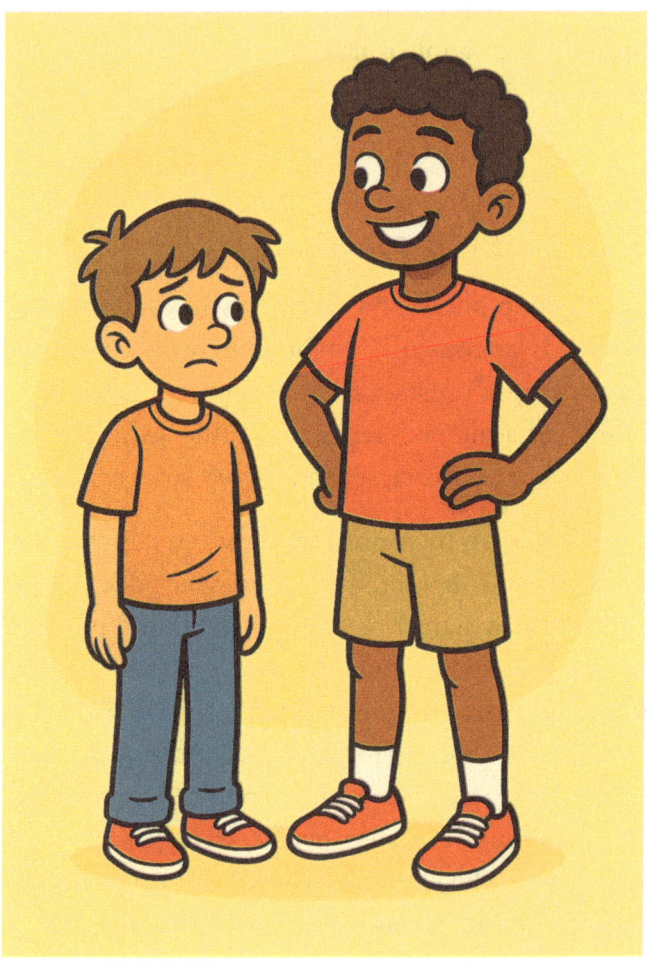

Worrying about being "too early" is normal, too. Maybe you're first to need deodorant or get armpit hair. Being ahead of the curve can feel just as odd as being behind. But your friends will catch up—everyone gets there, just not all at once.

When it comes to puberty, there's a wide range of normal. Some guys hit their growth spurts early, some much later, and most fall somewhere in between. I knew one group with boys who looked grown-up in fifth grade and others who stayed small until high school—by graduation, nobody could tell who grew first or last.

It can be tough not to compare yourself to others, especially when everyone seems obsessed with height, muscles, or shaving. But if you spend all your energy worrying about everyone else's changes, you'll miss out on what's cool about your own progress. Some changes, like getting stronger or more confident, come slowly. Others, like a new shoe size or deeper voice, seem to happen overnight.

If you start feeling down about being different, try tracking your own milestones. Keep a "Growth Journal." Jot down the firsts—new hair, voice changes, outgrowing your hoodie, or finally reaching that top shelf. Write about how these moments made you feel—excited, weird, proud, or even nervous. Every note is proof you're moving forward at your own pace.

If you ever get anxious about being different, remind yourself: "I'm on my own timeline, and that's okay." That's not just a cheesy saying—it's true. Everybody grows in their own way, and your journey doesn't need to match anyone else's for you to end up confident and strong.

Growth Journal Prompt

Tonight, or whenever you find a quiet minute, write down something unique about your growing-up story. Was there a surprising change? Did you feel happy, nervous, or both? If you prefer drawing, sketch what "growing at your own pace" looks like—even if it's just stick figures. You don't have to share it unless you want to.

Remember, every boy has his own timeline—even if it feels like your journey is in slow-mo or warp speed compared to everyone else. That's normal, and perfectly okay.

DEALING WITH EMBARRASSING MOMENTS—FROM VOICE CRACKS TO SPLITTING YOUR PANTS

Everyone faces embarrassing moments, especially during puberty, when everything seems to go wrong at the worst time. Maybe you slip in gym class and slide across the floor with everyone watching, your voice cracks in the middle of a speech, your jeans split as you run for the bus, or you realize your socks don't match during a big event. Even small things, like deodorant marks on your shirt, can feel like the end of the world. These moments sting because no one wants negative attention or to stand out!

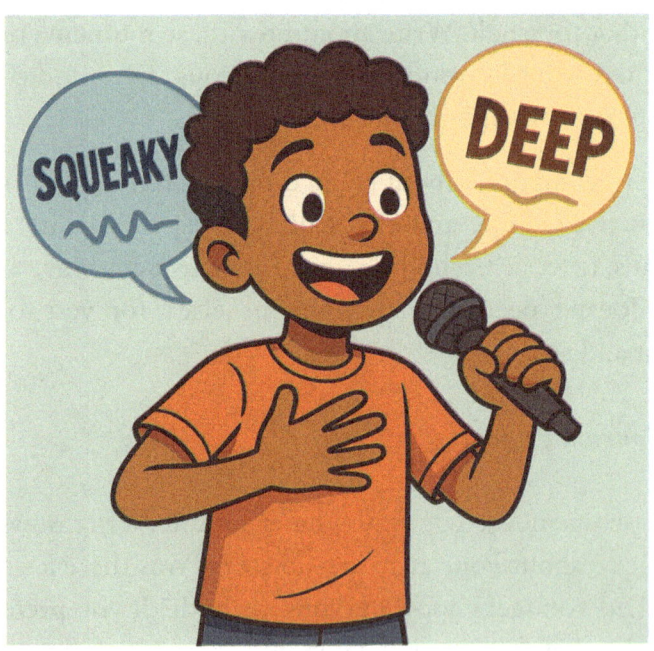

But you're not alone—everyone has similar stories, even if they don't admit it. One boy wore his shirt inside out all day and only noticed when someone pointed it out at lunch. Another, during a school play, cracked his voice so loudly that even teachers laughed —yet he got through the scene anyway. There's also the classic: ripping your pants in gym, then tying a sweatshirt around your waist and finishing strong.

Awkward things happen because your body is changing and your brain is learning to adjust. You can't prevent every embarrassing moment. The real challenge is how you react afterward. If your voice cracks or you trip up, laughing at yourself can make it less of a big deal. A quick joke—like, "Guess my pants wanted to be shorts!"—shows you're okay, which helps others move on as well.

If you get a rush of embarrassment and want to disappear, that's normal, too. In these moments, take a deep breath, remind yourself everyone's been there (even adults), and try to focus on what's next rather than what just happened. Breaking the tension with a joke or even saying, "Well, that was awkward," helps. If you're too embarrassed to speak, just nod and move on—most people forget about it quickly.

If embarrassment leads to ongoing teasing or people won't let it go, don't hesitate to reach out for help. Lots of adults have had their own awkward moments and will understand. After a rough day, talk to someone you trust, like:

- Parent or caregiver
- Grandparent
- Teacher or counselor
- Coach
- Older sibling
- Family friend

You can start with, "Has this ever happened to you?" or, "Can I tell you about something awkward?" Most people will share their own stories and help you realize you're not alone. Knowing others have survived similar moments makes your embarrassment feel smaller.

Some boys manage their awkward moments in creative ways. One kept a "Cringe List" on his phone as proof that bad moments fade over time—sometimes even becoming funny memories. Another boy drew comics of his embarrassing stories, like a voice squeak at the drive-thru or waving at someone who wasn't waving back. Seeing these moments as comics helped him recognize that what once felt like a disaster was actually just a funny story.

Self-kindness is key when you're embarrassed. Don't replay the moment endlessly in your head. Tell yourself, "It happens," or, "Next time will be better." Make up your own light-hearted phrase —like "Oops, puberty strikes again!"—as a reminder that these times pass.

If embarrassment keeps you from wanting to go to school or participate in activities, talk it over with someone you trust. Putting your experience into words can shrink it from huge to manageable. Remember: every grown-up has tripped at work or said the wrong thing in a meeting. They get it.

Finally, remember that no one is keeping score of your embarrassing moments but you. Everyone else is focused on their own worries. Awkward things happen to everyone while growing up, and they never last as long as they feel like they do, in the moment.

WHAT IF I DON'T WANT TO TALK?—PRIVACY, JOURNALS, AND FINDING TRUSTED ADULTS

Sometimes, you may not feel ready to talk about changes in your body or feelings. You might worry your thoughts are strange, too private, or hard to express. That's normal—many people prefer privacy at times, need more time to open up, or may not want to talk at all. Wanting to keep things to yourself is totally okay; it just means you're figuring things out your own way.

When you're not ready to talk, there are different ways to handle confusing thoughts or big feelings. Try jotting things down in a journal, notebook, or a phone note that's just for you. You can write what's happening, draw what's on your mind, or use shapes and stick figures if words are tough. Some boys write letters to their future selves about their struggles or hopes, or just scribble quick notes like, "I feel weird about my voice," or, "Why am I so angry?" These can stay private or be read later to see your growth. If regular writing feels too intense, use code words or comics. The goal is to get thoughts out of your head, even if nobody else sees them.

If you want to explore feelings without talking, try making a feelings chart using colors or emojis for different moods. Some people put sticky notes on the wall for each feeling and move them around through the week. You could keep a secret folder on your device with stories, songs, or pictures that match your mood. If you prefer movement, try kicking a soccer ball while thinking things over or go for a walk when you feel stuck. Any method that helps untangle your thoughts counts.

Even if you like privacy most of the time, it's helpful to know who you might talk to if you feel overwhelmed. Make a mental list of possible listeners—a coach, school counselor, youth pastor, aunt, older sibling, or a teacher who understands awkward stuff. Trusted adults aren't just parents, and the right person is whoever helps you feel safe and less judged.

When you're ready (even just a little), starting a conversation doesn't have to be a big deal. Simple openers help: "I have a weird question…" or "Something's bugging me but it's hard to say." If talking face-to-face is intimidating, try a note or text, like, "Can we talk later?" or give someone your written note to read first.

You don't need long speeches or special words—most adults remember puberty can feel private and weird. If your first try at sharing doesn't help, pick someone else. You only need to confide in the person who makes you feel comfortable, even if it's just a quick message about a tough day.

Some boys ask for advice through notes, leaving questions on the kitchen counter or under a door. Others use anonymous school apps to reach counselors. If drawing is easier, sketch your feelings and show someone instead of explaining.

Try prompts like writing a letter to your future self about what's hard now and what you hope improves: "Today was rough but hopefully next year I'll laugh about it." These letters help you look back later and see how things have changed.

Choosing privacy now doesn't mean you'll always want it. It's okay to change your mind—privacy isn't isolation, just what you need for the moment. If things get too heavy, remember that reaching out isn't weakness; it's self-care, like eating or sleeping.

No one gets things perfect the first time. If your first attempt at sharing feels awkward or doesn't help, it's okay to try again with someone else or a different approach. The right person will listen as you sort things out—even if all you need is a listening ear or someone to say, "That sounds tough." And if writing or keeping things private is what works best right now, that's perfectly fine too.

MYTH-BUSTER COMICS—PLAYGROUND RUMORS VS. REAL SCIENCE

You've probably come across some wild "facts" about puberty while hanging out with friends or scrolling on your phone—some are funny, others can make you worry. But most aren't true, so it's time for a Myth-Buster moment to sort out reality from playground gossip.

Imagine a comic: two kids chatting at their lockers. One goes, "Crack your knuckles and your hands will get huge!" The other says, "My uncle's been cracking his knuckles forever and his hands are normal." Comic solved: knuckle cracking does not make your hands grow. That's just one of many myths that sound believable but aren't backed by science.

Another classic: "Eating lots of spicy food makes you grow a mustache sooner." Picture a boy downing hot wings in front of a mirror, waiting for hair to magically sprout. The truth: spicy food has zero effect on how fast you grow facial hair; hormones are in charge of that, not hot sauce.

Then there's the wild myth: "Too many wet dreams and you'll run out of sperm." Imagine a superhero boy frantically checking his "sperm fuel gauge." Reality? Your body makes new sperm all the time and never "runs out." Wet dreams don't empty your supply, just like sneezing doesn't use up all your air.

Some rumors just get more bizarre. "If you're in puberty too long, you'll be stuck there forever." Visualize a kid trapped in a giant "puberty" cocoon while friends stroll by as adults. Not true—

everyone gets through puberty at their own pace; no one stays stuck forever.

False stories spread fast because they're funny or a little scary. Each year, you'll hear the same old ones: "Shave early and hair grows back thicker," or "Cracking your neck will make you taller." When you hear something like that, pause—does it make sense? Is it from someone reliable, like a doctor or teacher?

When in doubt, look for the "Real Talk" seal—science-based advice from people who actually know. Don't be fooled easily by playground experts! If something sounds weird, write it down and ask someone who knows, such as your school nurse or a parent. You could end up teaching friends the truth instead of passing along rumors.

Let's take another favorite: "If you're short now, you'll always be short." Picture a small boy with tall parents joking, "We were tiny too!" Growth happens on everyone's own timetable, not by one simple rule. Or, "Skip deodorant once and everyone will notice." Imagine a boy sniffing his armpit in class while everyone else is busy reading. The reality: missing deodorant is no big deal for a day. Good hygiene matters for confidence, but no one is perfect all the time.

Don't let rumors make you embarrassed or anxious about things that are perfectly normal or out of your control. Myths often come from people just trying to be funny or act like they know everything. It's fine to laugh, but smarter to check before believing—and definitely before repeating.

When you hear something wacky like, "Drinking coffee makes your voice deeper," jot it down and ask an adult. You'll be surprised how many tall tales fall apart with a little research.

Everyone deals with weird stories like these growing up. The key is not letting them make puberty scarier or more confusing than it needs to be. Rely on science, keep asking questions, and use your sense of humor.

As this chapter wraps up, remember: It's normal to get mixed up by the wild things people say about puberty, but now you know how to separate fact from fiction—and help others do the same. Continue to question and search for genuine answers. Up next: how to be a confident guy who treats himself and everyone else with respect and kindness.

8

CONFIDENCE, CONSENT & KINDNESS—GROWING INTO THE BEST VERSION OF YOU

WHAT DOES "BEING A MAN" REALLY MEAN? (SPOILER: THERE'S NO ONE WAY)

Who decides what "being a man" actually means? Society acts like there's a hidden rulebook, full of sayings like, "Real men don't cry" or "Man up!" Movies often show guys as tough and silent, never discussing their feelings. Maybe you've felt pressured to act this way, even though it feels uncomfortable. Here's the truth: there is no single way to be a man. If only someone had said that earlier! Being a man isn't about hiding your feelings or pretending you're emotionless—it's about being true to who you are.

Many old ideas about boys just don't fit anymore. Some people still think boys should always be tough, fearless, or into sports. But in reality, you get to decide what kind of man you want to be.

Some of the most interesting guys I know are nothing alike. When I asked a few boys and men what being a man means to them, Ethan, an eighth grader, said, "Being a man is trying your best to do the right thing, even when it's hard." Mr. Ramirez, a father from my church, said, "It means showing up for my family and listening when they need me." My friend Andre, a cellist, (that's a person who plays the cello) said, "It means owning your weirdness and helping others feel welcome." Notice: none of them talked about muscles or pretending they never cry.

Look around and you'll see role models everywhere—guys who break stereotypes every day.

There's Mr. Evans, a nurse who's gentle and makes kids laugh even when they're scared. Jake is a stay-at-home dad who runs an awesome Lego club and can braid his daughter's hair in no time. Keith is a professional gamer who talks openly about coping with stress and anxiety, proving you can be competitive and still talk about your feelings. Marcus, a classical musician, uses music to express his emotions, from joy to sadness. Gabe organizes fundraisers and stands up for bullied kids—he's an activist who leads with compassion.

What do all these men share? Their strength looks different from old stereotypes. Sometimes strength is helping someone else, standing up for what's right, or simply not giving up. Maybe you feel strong when you tackle a tough math problem or admit a mistake to a friend. Or, maybe it's letting yourself cry rather than pretending you're always fine.

Reflection: Your Own Definition of Manhood

Think about the men and boys you admire—dads, grandpas, teachers, coaches, older brothers, or friends. What stands out about them? Write down three qualities you admire. Maybe they listen, are patient, tell jokes when you're sad, fix bikes, or cook pancakes. Which of these do you want for yourself? List them.

CONFIDENCE, CONSENT & KINDNESS—GROWING INTO TH... | 135

There are so many ways to be strong that don't involve being tough or big. Some examples:

- Standing up for someone being picked on
- Admitting mistakes and apologizing
- Asking for help
- Practicing to improve
- Comforting a struggling friend
- Telling the truth, even when it's tough
- Laughing at yourself after a mistake

Affirmation Exercise: 3 Things

3 Things	
I am good at …	I like about me …
①	①
②	②
③	③

It's easy to feel pressure to act how others think boys should. But you choose who you want to be. When you hear, "man up" or "boys don't cry," you can say, "Everyone has feelings—it's okay to show them." If someone teases you for being caring instead of "tough," just reply, "Being a good friend is just as important as being tough." You don't need to argue—just keep being yourself.

Being a man is about kindness, honesty, and courage—not just acting cool or hiding your emotions. Every boy creates his own story. Yours can be filled with music, science, sports, art, jokes, or listening—whatever feels right for you. There are as many paths to manhood as there are boys in the world. Choose the one that makes you proud of who you're becoming.

CONSENT BASICS—RESPECTING BOUNDARIES AND SAYING NO

Consent isn't just for big issues you see on TV—it's something you use every day. At its core, consent means asking someone before doing something that might affect them, and waiting for their answer. It's simply saying, "Is this okay with you?" and truly listening. If the answer is yes, you go ahead. If it's no—or if the person seems unsure or uncomfortable—you stop, no questions asked. There's no secret code or guessing; you just ask and pay attention.

Think about when someone grabs your stuff without asking or gives you an unexpected hug. Sometimes it's fine, sometimes it's uncomfortable. You have every right to say, "No thanks," or "Not right now," and that should be respected—just as you respect others. For example, if you want to borrow your friend's game, you ask first: "Hey, can I use this?" If you want to hug your grandma, you check: "Do you want a hug?" She might say yes, or maybe, "Not now, my back hurts." Both are totally okay.

Consent can show up anywhere: sharing snacks at lunch, joining a game at recess, taking pictures at a party, or posting something online. You might say, "Want some chips?" or "Can I invite you to our group?" Asking first makes everyone more comfortable—no one feels forced or left out, and everyone knows their feelings matter.

Often, answers aren't just yes or no. A friend might shrug, say "Maybe later," look away, or not say much. That isn't a yes. When in doubt, wait, or check again another time. People can always change their minds, even after saying yes—that's their right. Consent isn't a one-time thing.

Here's how to recognize consent: A real yes sounds clear and positive—"Yeah!" "Sure!" or a happy thumbs-up. A no sounds like "No thanks," or "Not right now." Uncertain answers—"I don't know," "Maybe," or silence—mean you don't have a clear yes. Don't push if someone looks uncomfortable or quiet—they might not want to say no out loud.

Getting and giving consent is about respect and paying attention to both words and body language. If you ask to join a game and hear, "We're full right now," don't argue or beg—just accept it. If you invite someone to hang out and they say they're busy, answer, "No worries!" People notice when you respect their choices.

It's not always easy to say no, especially if you don't want to upset anyone, but your comfort matters. It's fine to say, "No thanks, I'd rather not," or "Not today." Honesty isn't rude. If someone's upset by your no, that's on them—real friends don't pressure you.

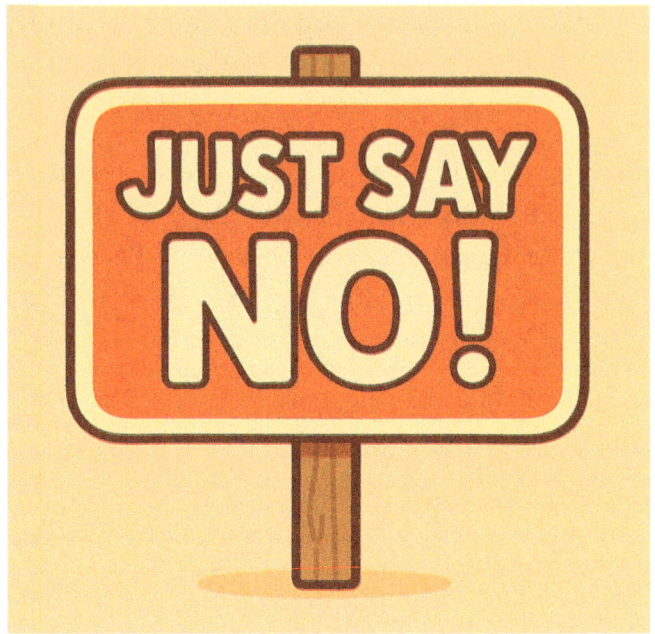

Online boundaries matter as much as in-person ones. Before posting a group photo or tagging someone, ask: "Is it okay if I post this?" Not everyone wants everything shared. If someone asks you to take something down, do it without a fuss.

Looking out for friends is also important. If you see someone looking uncomfortable or unable to say no, check on them later: "Hey, was that okay for you?" Sometimes people need support to speak up.

You have the right to your own boundaries—big and small—and so does everyone else. Respecting consent strengthens friendships and builds trust. The more you practice asking for and respecting consent, the easier it becomes to be honest and kind.

Quick Guide: How Consent Sounds in Daily Life

- **Friend**: "Want to share my fries?"
    - **You:** "Yes please!" or "No thanks."
- Someone tries to borrow your book:
    - **You**: "I'd rather keep it today."
- Group wants you to join a game:
    - **You**: "I'll watch this time."
- Friend wants your photo for social media:
    - **You:** "Sure!" or "Can we wait?"

Learning these responses and questions keeps things clear and fair for everyone. No one gets it perfect every time—it takes practice. But asking and listening shows respect, and that's something people will remember.

BEING KIND TO YOURSELF—HANDLING MISTAKES AND SELF-DOUBT

Nobody gets through growing up without stumbling. Even the most "together" kid in your class makes mistakes, feels nervous, or wonders if he's good enough. Some days, you might feel like you just can't do anything right. That's normal, especially when so many things are changing inside and out. I remember when my own son failed a math test in sixth grade. He was so sure he was the only one who messed up. He came home, slammed his backpack down, and said, "I'm just dumb." My heart broke a little, but I told him the truth—messing up is part of learning. He didn't believe me right away, but over time, he saw that one test didn't say who he was.

Everyone feels self-doubt sometimes. Maybe you missed a shot that could have won the game. Maybe you forgot your lines in a play or blanked on a quiz. Sometimes it feels like everyone's watching, waiting for you to mess up again. But here's the real deal: mistakes do not define you. They're just events, little blips on your radar. The important part is what you do after. When things go wrong, give yourself a second to pause. Take a breath—really breathe in, then let it out slow. Think about what happened. Ask yourself, "What can I learn from this?" Then, when you're ready, try again. You don't have to fix everything at once. Sometimes the bravest thing you can do is just show up and try.

I know it sounds easy for grown-ups to say "don't be so hard on yourself." But that voice inside your head—the one that calls you "loser," "weird," or "not good enough"—isn't telling the truth. Everyone has a "mean voice" in their mind sometimes, but you can answer back with kinder words. Here's a quick look at how that might work:

Mean Voice	Kind Voice
I always make mistakes	Everyone makes mistakes
Nobody likes me	Some people do like me
I'm not smart enough	I can learn and get better with practice
Why even try?	Trying brings growth and understanding

If you notice your thoughts getting mean, challenge them. Is what you're thinking really true? Or are you being harder on yourself than you'd be to a friend? Talk to yourself the way you'd talk to someone you care about.

One of the best ways to beat self-doubt is to celebrate effort, not just wins. It's easy to look at the scoreboard or the grade on your paper and feel like that's all people see. However, what matters most is that you continue to show up and put in the work. If you practiced your speech even though you felt scared, that's a win. If you apologized after snapping at someone, that counts. If you tried out for a team and didn't make it but learned something new, that's real progress.

When you mess up (and you will), remember this: one mistake doesn't wipe out all your good days or erase all your hard work. You're allowed to have off days and second tries. Everyone around you—parents, teachers, friends—has felt the sting of failure before. What sets people apart isn't never falling down; it's getting back up with honesty and courage.

So the next time self-doubt creeps in or you trip over your own feet (literally or not), remember to pause, breathe, look for what you can learn, and try again. Talk back to those harsh thoughts with something kinder and truer. Keep track of the times you put yourself out there or learned from something tough. That's how confidence grows—not from being perfect, but from being real and never giving up on yourself.

SHOWING RESPECT ONLINE AND OFFLINE—BUILDING A POSITIVE REPUTATION

Respect is bigger than raising your hand in class or saying "please" at the dinner table. It stretches into everything you do—on the field, in the locker room, on your phone, and even when you're gaming with friends you might never meet face-to-face. What you say and do in person leaves an impression, but what you post or share online can stick around much longer. Imagine this: would you tell someone their haircut looks weird if they were standing right in front of you? If not, why would you type it in a group chat? That screen might feel like a shield, but there's still a real person on the other side.

Think about your day at school. Respect shows up when you listen without talking over others, or when you thank your teacher for helping you after class. Maybe it's holding the door for someone who's carrying too much, or cheering for a teammate even after a tough game. In sports, being a good sport means shaking hands, not bragging, and giving credit where it's due. When someone scores a goal—even if it's not you—you can say, "Nice shot!" or "Great try!" That little bit of kindness sticks with people.

Now, flip to digital life. It's easy to forget how fast things move online. A meme about a classmate might seem funny for a second, but it can hurt for days. You get to choose whether to laugh along, ignore it, or speak up. Not laughing at a mean meme is a kind choice. If you see someone posting an embarrassing photo or a rumor, you can send a private message: "Maybe don't share that—it could hurt them." Even something as small as giving a compliment on someone's art in a group chat ("That drawing is awesome!") makes digital spaces more positive.

Before you hit send, take a beat. Ask yourself, "Would I want this said about me?" If the answer is no, it's probably not worth sharing. Try this quick checklist before posting:

Post with Pride—5-Second Kindness Check

- Would I say this to someone's face?
- Would I want my grandma or coach to see this?
- Is this kind? Helpful? True?
- Could this embarrass or hurt someone?

- Will I be okay if this pops up years from now?

If you hesitate on any of these, it's smart to pause. You don't have to post everything you think or see. The internet can feel private, but screenshots and shares make things travel fast. Stuff that seems small now—an angry comment during a game, a silly post from a sleepover—can show up years later when you least expect it.

Let me tell you about Tyler. He once posted a silly video of himself and some friends dancing in pajamas. Years later, that goofy clip popped up when he was running for student council. Instead of making him look bad, everyone remembered how funny and kind he was in that video—he owned it and even got more votes! On the flip side, Josh found out the hard way that teasing friends in a group chat can backfire. Someone screenshotted his messages and shared them outside the group. It caused a lot of drama at school, and he ended up having to apologize to more people than he could count.

It's never too late to clean up your online footprint. Go back through your old posts or messages—if anything feels mean, embarrassing, or just not like you anymore, delete it. Set your social media to private if you want more control over who sees what. Change old passwords if needed. If something bad gets out of control, ask an adult for help—you don't have to fix it alone.

Gaming is another place where respect matters. Trash talk might be part of some games, but there's a line between fun and mean. If someone misses a move or loses connection, don't pile on insults. Instead, say something supportive: "You'll get it next time" or "It happens." Good teammates remember how you treat them as much as how many points you score.

Your reputation—how people see and remember you—is shaped by these choices every single day. Small acts of respect build trust and make people want to be around you. You want to be known as someone who stands up for others, keeps secrets safe, and doesn't spread drama just for laughs.

When in doubt, ask yourself if what you're about to do will build someone up or tear them down. Respect isn't about being perfect —it's about learning, trying again when you mess up, and caring how your actions make others feel. Both in real life and online, kindness has power. It makes people feel seen and safe, including yourself.

THE TOP 10 AWKWARD QUESTIONS—ANSWERED WITH HONESTY & HUMOR

Ever find your brain saving the weirdest, cringiest questions for late at night or in the middle of class? If you're wondering, "Am I the only one who thinks this?"—you're definitely not alone.

These are the questions most boys never say out loud, but everyone thinks about. I've heard these whispered many times, scribbled on anonymous notes, and even grown-ups remember wondering the same stuff (and laughing or cringing about puberty later). Here's the real talk, no filter—straight answers to those embarrassing questions, with some humor (because laughing makes it all less awkward).

"Why do I sometimes wake up with 'morning wood'?"

Waking up with an erection—morning wood—is completely normal. Whether you had wild dreams or dreamt about pancakes, it's just hormones acting up during sleep. It happens to most guys almost every morning, others less often. Needing to pee can make it last longer. Just give it a bit, use the bathroom, and move on.

"Is it normal for one testicle to hang lower than the other?"

Totally normal. Most guys have one testicle that hangs lower or feels bigger (usually the left). It's just how you're built—like how your ears aren't identical. Only worry if there's pain, swelling, or a sudden change; then, talk to an adult or doctor.

"What's up with random erections in class?"

Bodies are unpredictable! You can be reading about volcanoes and —bam—random erection. It's not about what you're thinking. Puberty just has your body running test programs. If it happens, cover with a book or hoodie until it goes away. Most people don't notice or care, and by lunchtime, no one remembers.

"Can you start puberty and then stop?"

Puberty isn't an on/off switch. Sometimes changes come quickly, then pause for a while. That's normal! Puberty takes years, not weeks—stuff is happening behind the scenes even if you can't see it.

"Why do I sweat so much—even when I'm not hot?"

Blame hormones! Sweat glands go wild during puberty. You might sweat more, even just worrying about awkward moments. Showers and deodorant help, but know everyone your age is sweating buckets—even if they pretend they aren't.

"Is it okay if I cry more than I used to?"

Yes. Puberty amps up your emotions, making crying more common. It's not a sign of weakness—it just means your brain is processing new feelings and stress. Even grown-ups cry, so you're not alone. Letting feelings out is healthier than bottling them up.

"What if I never get an Adam's apple?"

Not everyone gets a big, noticeable Adam's apple. Some are hardly visible, others more obvious. Both are normal—it doesn't say anything about how mature you are.

"Is it normal to feel shy about changing in front of others?"

Absolutely. Most boys feel awkward in locker rooms or at sleepovers and want to change quickly or hang on to their towel. Some may look confident, but many feel just as weird inside. Over time, you'll get more comfortable or figure out tricks that make it easier.

"Can you be too young or too old for puberty?"

Puberty for boys usually starts between ages 8 and 14. Starting earlier or later can both be normal. If you're over 15 or 16 and nothing's happening, check with a doctor just to be sure.

"Why do I sometimes feel super confident, then suddenly not?"

Welcome to the puberty roller coaster! One day you're confident; the next you're not. Mood swings are normal—they're from changing brain chemistry and stress. It won't always be this wild, and remember: everyone else is in the same boat.

Growing up, I once asked my brother if he had these questions as a kid. He admitted he thought he was the only "freak." Turns out, nobody's alone in wondering this stuff. If you have random questions, jot them down in a notebook or on your phone, and ask a trusted adult, doctor, or coach, or search for good answers in books or reliable websites for teens. Curiosity is part of growing up, and embarrassment can't stand up to honest questions and good information.

YOUR NEXT LIFE-CHAPTER—GROWING UP WITH CONFIDENCE AND PRIDE

You've already come a long way. Puberty is full of ups and downs—and plenty of surprises. It can feel like a wild roller coaster with no map, but you've navigated changing bodies, new feelings, tricky social moments, and lots of questions. In all the confusion, it's easy to forget how much you've grown. But here's the real truth: growing up is about taking charge of your own story, not letting someone else tell it. You choose how to handle tough moments. You choose kindness—not because you have to, but because you know it matters. With every step, whether you're standing up for yourself, helping someone, or learning from a setback, you're shaping the person you'll become.

Remember, there's only one you. No one else shares your exact mix of quirks, skills, dreams, or sense of humor. On hard days, or when you feel out of place, it can be easy to forget that being unique is your superpower. Just by being yourself, you always bring something new to every space you enter—whether it's a classroom, team, or even a group chat. It's not about being the loudest or most popular. It's about being genuine, especially when things feel uncertain.

As you move forward, think about what comes next. Puberty isn't your whole story—it's just one part. What's something new you want to try next? Maybe a new skateboard trick, speaking up in class, joining a club, starting to draw, cook, or run. Pick one thing—big or small—and write it somewhere you'll see. Choose a goal that excites you, or even makes you a little nervous. That's where real growth happens.

Of course, you'll still have days when your confidence dips—that's normal. Everyone faces tough patches. When it happens, try these three quick steps: get active for a few minutes, talk to someone who cares, and remember a past success, even a small one. Remind yourself of a time something seemed impossible and now it's easy. That memory can help you get through the rough patch.

As you grow, you also have the chance to help others. Being a role model doesn't mean being perfect. It means sharing what you've learned, maybe with younger friends, siblings, or classmates struggling with their own awkward moments. If someone feels nervous about growing up, let them know they aren't alone—a kind word or sharing a tip that helped you can make all the difference.

Affirmation Exercise & Growth Tracker

Here's a challenge: this week, help someone younger who seems stressed about growing up. Maybe they're worried about gym class or their changing voice. Tell them something that helped you, or just listen if they need to talk. If you want, share your favorite tip from this book—maybe even with an adult who could use a reminder, too.

Growing up means you'll make mistakes and learn on the go. Some days you'll feel unstoppable; others, you'll want to hide under your blanket. Both are normal! What matters is that you keep moving forward, keep laughing when things get awkward, and keep believing that being yourself is always enough.

You are writing your story every day, even on uneventful days. Each choice matters. Each act of kindness counts. The world needs people who are real, who try new things, and who support others.

Just as one chapter ends and another begins, remember: puberty won't last forever, but the confidence and kindness you build now will always be with you. Take pride in your journey, and get excited for what's next—there's so much more to discover.

Stay true to yourself—the next part of your story is yours to create.

CONCLUSION

Hey there. If you're reading this, I just want to start by telling you how proud I am of you. Seriously. You picked up a book about puberty and stuck with it. That takes guts. I know it's not as fun as playing games or scrolling funny videos, but you did it anyway. That says a lot about your curiosity and your courage. I've always believed that asking questions—even the weird or awkward ones—means you're brave and ready to grow. So, high-five to you for showing up for yourself.

When I wrote this book, I wanted it to feel like a chat with someone who really gets it. Not a boring lecture. Not another class you have to sit through. I wanted to give you honest answers, some laughs, and a reminder that you're not alone in any of this. Think of this book as the friend who sits next to you on the bus, the coach who gives you a thumbs up, or maybe the big sibling who tells you the truth (without making it weird). My hope is that you felt supported, seen, and maybe even a little more chill about all the changes you're going through.

Let's take a quick trip down memory lane and remember what you've just learned. You started by finding out what puberty actually means—and why everyone's timeline is a bit different. Maybe your voice cracked at the dinner table, or you noticed hair in new places where it wasn't before. You learned that all these changes are normal, even if they don't happen at the same time as your friends. We talked about growth spurts, new smells, pimples, and how your body might feel like it's running its own wild show for a while.

We tackled hygiene head-on. You got real tips for dealing with body odor, showers, clothes, and even those stubborn zits. No shame, just real talk.

Then, we dove into feelings—the good, the bad, and the "why do I want to yell into my pillow right now?" kind. Mood swings, anxiety, wanting to be alone, and talking to yourself kindly. You learned that tough days don't last, and there's always a way to bounce back.

You got advice for friendships, too—how to find your squad, handle teasing, deal with peer pressure, stand up for others, and recover when you're left out. You learned that being a good friend and standing up for yourself is a real superpower. And you saw that even online, you can be a force for kindness and respect.

We covered how to fuel your body—what to eat, why water matters, why sleep is your secret weapon, and how moving your body helps you feel better. We busted myths about lifting weights, and gave you tricks for getting through energy slumps without reaching for a sugar bomb.

You even got the answers to the questions nobody wants to ask out loud. Erections, wet dreams, embarrassing moments, and all the stuff that makes most people squirm. You learned that every question is welcome, and nothing about your body is too strange or weird to talk about.

Most of all, I hope you remember this: There is no one "right" way to go through puberty. Your story is unique. Your body, your feelings, your timeline—they are all yours. Some things will be easy. Some things will be awkward. Sometimes you'll feel on top of the world, and sometimes you'll wish you could hit the fast-forward button. All of that is normal. Really!

Taking care of your body—showering, brushing teeth, eating well, moving, sleeping—these things aren't just chores. They are ways to build confidence. They help you feel ready to face whatever comes next, even if it's a day when nothing goes right.

Feelings are part of the deal, too. Mood swings, worry, sadness, excitement—they are all signs that you're growing and learning. And it's okay to talk about them. Or write them down. Or ask for help when you need it.

Friendships matter. So does standing up for yourself and others. You don't have to be the loudest or the most popular. Just be the person who listens, includes others, and tries to do the right thing. That's real strength.

Here's what I hope you remember most: Asking questions is brave. Speaking up when you need help is strong. Being kind to yourself and others is the best superpower you can have. Respect, honesty, and kindness will take you far—at school, online, in your squad, and everywhere you go.

I know it can feel scary or awkward to talk about puberty. Maybe you still have questions. That's okay! Keep asking. Find trusted adults—parents, grandparents, teachers, coaches, counselors—or write your thoughts down if talking is tough. You are not supposed to figure it all out on your own. There are always people who want to help, even when it doesn't feel that way.

Most of all, please remember that your differences are something to celebrate. Whether you're tall, short, loud, quiet, sporty, artsy, or anything in between—you have value. The world needs you, just as you are. Your story matters. You are fearfully and wonderfully made.

Now, here's my challenge for you: Take one step today. Try out a new hygiene habit. Send a message to a friend who might feel left out. Start a journal, or share something you learned from this book with someone else. Every little action counts. You don't have to do it all at once. Just keep moving forward, one real step at a time.

Growing-up is a wild ride. It's full of changes, questions, and sometimes a few epic fails. But it's also full of new strengths, new friends, and new chances to be the best version of yourself. Puberty is just one chapter. There's so much more ahead for you. You're never alone—no matter how weird, awkward, or confusing things get.

I believe in you. I'm cheering you on. Thanks for letting me be part of your journey. And don't forget—confidence comes from knowing, caring, and being kind. You've got this. Now go out there and keep growing, learning, and being awesome—just as you are.

- DebbieAnn

THANK YOU FOR READING! NOW, LET'S HELP OTHERS TOGETHER

You've made it through *The Essential Boy's Guide to Puberty & Body Changes*—congratulations! Armed with the knowledge and confidence from this guide, you're ready to navigate puberty like a pro.

Now, you have the chance to pay it forward.

By leaving an honest **review on Amazon**, you're not just sharing your thoughts—you're helping other boys, parents, teachers, and even grandparents discover this guide. Your feedback could be the reason someone else gains the tools to handle this journey with confidence and courage.

Your Voice Matters

When you share your experience, you're making a real difference. Your insights might help someone overcome fears, embrace changes, and feel more prepared for this important stage of life.

It Only Takes a Moment

Click below to leave your review and share how this book made a difference for you or your family:

Scan the QR code to Leave Your Review on Amazon

Thank You for Being Part of This Journey

Your support helps keep this essential guide alive and available for those who need it most. I can't thank you enough for your kindness and generosity in sharing your thoughts.

Together, we're making puberty a little less scary and a lot more manageable—for everyone. With heartfelt gratitude,

- DebbieAnn Lewis

GLOSSARY OF TERMS

Puberty can feel overwhelming with so many new things to learn, but don't worry—you're not alone! This glossary explains important words you'll see in this guide. If you're unsure about a term, come back to this page anytime to find its meaning.

A

Acne - Small bumps or pimples that can appear on your skin, especially your face, during puberty because of hormonal changes.
Adolescence - The stage between being a child and an adult when your body and mind are growing and changing.

B

Balance - Learning to manage school, friendships, family, and self-care in a healthy way.
Blemishes - Small marks, spots, or imperfections on the skin, often caused by clogged pores, excess oil, or bacteria. They are common during puberty due to hormonal changes.

C

Crush - A strong feeling of admiration or affection, often for someone you find interesting, attractive, or fun to be around. For middle schoolers, a crush is usually an innocent and exciting feeling that might make you want to spend more time with or think about that person a lot.
Confidence - Believing in yourself and your abilities, even when facing challenges or changes.
Cultural - Customs, traditions, and practices that vary by region, family, or group, including those related to puberty and periods.

D

Diet - The food you eat every day, which can affect how you feel during puberty and your period. Eating balanced meals helps your body stay healthy.

E

Ejaculation – When semen (a mix of sperm and fluids) comes out of the penis, usually during a wet dream or while masturbating.

Emotions - Feelings like happiness, sadness, anger, or excitement, which can be stronger during puberty because of changing hormones.

Erection – When the penis gets hard and stands up on its own. This happens when more blood flows into it. Erections can happen when you're thinking about something exciting, feeling nervous, or even for no reason at all—especially during puberty. It's totally normal and nothing to be embarrassed about.

F

Fatigue - Feeling very tired, which can happen before or during your period.

G

Glands - Small parts of your body that release hormones to help with growth and other changes.

Growing-Up - The process of maturing physically, emotionally, and mentally as you transition from a child to a young adult.

H

Hormones - Chemicals in your body that act as messengers, helping your body grow and change during puberty.

Hygiene - Keeping yourself clean and healthy.

I

Imbalance - When your hormones or emotions feel "off," which is normal during puberty.

M

Masturbation – When someone touches their own private parts for pleasure. It's a normal and private thing that some people do as they get older. Not everyone chooses to do it, and that's okay too. It's important to understand what feels right for you, respect your body, and know that this is a personal topic.

Mood Swings - Quick changes in how you feel, like going from happy to sad, caused by hormones.

N

Natural - Approaching puberty and self-care in a way that feels comfortable and true to yourself.

Nocturnal Emission (Wet Dream) – When semen comes out of the penis during sleep. It usually happens without you knowing.

P

Penis – The part of a boy's body that's used to pee and, later, to help make babies.

Puberty – The stage when your body starts changing from a kid into a teenager. It includes things like growing hair, voice changes, and growth spurts.

R

Romance - A special emotional connection or feeling of affection between two people, often involving admiration, kindness, and a desire to spend time together. For middle schoolers, it might mean having a crush or enjoying the company of someone who makes you feel happy and valued.

S

Scrotum – The pouch of skin that holds the testicles (balls). It hangs below the penis.

Semen – A fluid that contains sperm. It comes out of the penis during ejaculation.

Sperm - Male reproductive cells that are essential for fertilization. They are produced in the testes and can join with a female's egg to create a pregnancy.

T

Testicles (or Testes) – Two round organs in the scrotum that make sperm and testosterone.

Testosterone – The main male hormone that causes body changes during puberty, like voice deepening and muscle growth.

V

Voice Cracks – When your voice suddenly gets high or squeaky while it's changing. It's a normal part of voice deepening.

W

Wellness - Feeling healthy and balanced in your body and mind.

Wet Dream – Another name for a nocturnal emission. It's when ejaculation happens while you're asleep.

Z

Zits - Another word for pimples or spots that may appear during puberty.

REFERENCES

Puberty: Tanner Stages for Boys and Girls https://my.clevelandclinic.org/health/body/puberty

Stages of Puberty: A Guide for Males and Females - Healthline https://www.healthline.com/health/parenting/stages-of-puberty

How to talk to boys about puberty https://www.uclahealth.org/news/article/how-talk-boys-about-puberty

Common Myths About Pubertal Development https://www.aafp.org/pubs/afp/issues/2000/0915/p1406.html

Puberty: Tanner Stages for Boys and Girls https://my.clevelandclinic.org/health/body/puberty

Puberty: Adolescent Male https://www.hopkinsmedicine.org/health/wellness-and-prevention/puberty-adolescent-male

Why Is My Voice Changing? (for Teens) | Nemours KidsHealth https://kidshealth.org/en/teens/voice-changing.html#

13 tips for managing teen acne https://www.mayoclinichealthsystem.org/hometown-health/speaking-of-health/tips-for-managing-teen-acne

Hygiene: pre-teens and teenagers https://raisingchildren.net.au/pre-teens/healthy-lifestyle/hygiene-dental-care/hygiene-pre-teens-teens

Discussing Body Odor with Tweens and Choosing the Right ... https://www.pittsburghparent.com/discussing-body-odor-with-tweens-and-choosing-the-right-deodorant/#

Preteens and skincare: What parents should know - CHOC https://health.choc.org/preteens-and-skincare-what-parents-should-know/

How To Practice Good Oral Hygiene With Braces https://www.colgate.com/en-us/oral-health/kids-oral-care/how-to-practice-oral-hygiene-with-braces

Puberty: Tanner Stages for Boys and Girls https://my.clevelandclinic.org/health/body/puberty

Wheel of Emotions (Children) | Worksheet https://www.therapistaid.com/therapy-worksheet/wheel-of-emotions-children

25 Growth Mindset Activities To Inspire Confidence in Kids https://www.weareteachers.com/growth-mindset/

What to Do (and Not Do) When Children Are Anxious https://childmind.org/article/what-to-do-and-not-do-when-children-are-anxious/

8 ways to help your middle-schooler connect with other kids https://www.understood.

org/en/articles/8-ways-to-help-your-middle-schooler-connect-with-other-kids

How to Help your Child with Teasing https://www.speechandlanguagekids.com/kid-sounds-funny-insults-totally-respond/

How to Handle Peer Pressure https://kidshealth.org/en/kids/peer-pressure.html

Help Kids Fight Cyberbullying and Other Mean Online Behavior https://www.commonsense.org/education/family-tips/k-12-cyberbullying-digital-drama-and-hate-speech

Healthy food for pre-teens and teenagers: the 5 food groups https://raisingchildren.net.au/teens/healthy-lifestyle/daily-food-guides/nutrition-healthy-food-teens

Why is Hydration Important in Children https://copakids.com/child-healthcare-news/why-hydration-is-crucial-for-children/

Strength training: OK for kids? https://www.mayoclinic.org/healthy-lifestyle/tween-and-teen-health/in-depth/strength-training/art-20047758

School-age and pre-teen sleep: what to expect https://raisingchildren.net.au/pre-teens/healthy-lifestyle/sleep/school-age-sleep

Okay, well: 3 tricky questions young people often ask, and ... https://www.sexeducationaustralia.com.au/okay-well-3-tricky-questions-young-people-often-ask-and-how-to-answer-them/

What Are Wet Dreams? (for Teens) https://kidshealth.org/en/teens/expert-wet-dreams.html

Parenting children through puberty and adolescence https://www.betterhealth.vic.gov.au/health/healthyliving/Parenting-children-through-puberty#

Puberty myths your child needs debunked https://www.sexeducationaustralia.com.au/puberty-myths-your-child-needs-debunked/

Male Role Models: A Complete Guide on Positive ... https://mensgroup.com/male-role-models/

Consent at Every Age | Harvard Graduate School of Education https://www.gse.harvard.edu/ideas/usable-knowledge/18/12/consent-every-age

Resilience guide for parents and teachers https://www.apa.org/topics/resilience/guide-parents-teachers

DigCit Curriculum | Common Sense Education https://www.commonsense.org/education/digital-citizenship/curriculum

Made in the USA
Coppell, TX
10 March 2026

73146482R00095